Diseases of the Eye - Novel Investigations and Treatments

Edited by Felicia M. Ferreri

Published in London, United Kingdom

Diseases of the Eye - Novel Investigations and Treatments
http://dx.doi.org/10.5772/intechopen.1004495
Edited by Felicia M. Ferreri

Contributors
Aparajita Baruah, Benchu Feng, Cristina Irigoyen, Duo Xu, Faisal Aljassar, Fatemeh Naghshnejad, Fereshteh Karamali, Fuliang Li, Gulzhiyan Arzhimatova, Ke Mao, Leila Satarian, Ling Ai, Maryam Alsamhan, Maryam Bemanalizadeh, Mathew Shemiakin, Pamela Ríos, Reyhaneh Sadat Mousavi, Sangeetha Sreenivasa Pai, Sonjukta Borborah, Surya Prakash Goud Ponnam, Vahid Mansouri, Yunyun Wang, Zhilong Yang

First published in London, United Kingdom, 2025 by IntechOpen
IntechOpen is the global imprint of INTECHOPEN LIMITED, registered in England and Wales, registration number: 11086078, 167-169 Great Portland Street, London, W1W 5PF, United Kingdom

For EU product safety concerns: IN TECH d.o.o., Prolaz Marije Krucifikse Kozulić 3, 51000 Rijeka, Croatia, info@intechopen.com or visit our website at intechopen.com.

British Library Cataloguing-in-Publication Data
A catalogue record for this book is available from the British Library

Diseases of the Eye - Novel Investigations and Treatments
Edited by Felicia M. Ferreri
p. cm.
Print ISBN 978-1-83634-218-2
Online ISBN 978-1-83634-217-5
eBook (PDF) ISBN 978-1-83634-219-9

If disposing of this product, please recycle the paper responsibly.

Meet the editor

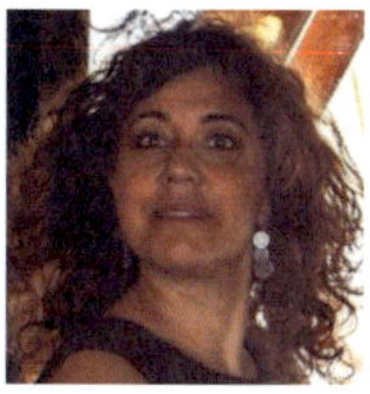

Felicia M. Ferreri graduated *magna cum laude* from the University of Messina in Italy in 1998 and completed her ophthalmology residency at the Policlinico Universitario in Messina in 2002. She then undertook internships at the Cornea Section of San Raffaele Hospital in Milan and the Paediatric Ophthalmology Diseases Section of Careggi Hospital in Florence. She undertook research placements at the Hospital Virgen del Rocío in Seville, the Hospital San Carlos in Madrid, the Royal Bolton Hospital in Manchester, and the Universidade Fluminense in Rio de Janeiro. She has served as a co-investigator on numerous national and international clinical trials. Since 2002, she has been an Assistant Professor of Ophthalmology at the University of Messina. Her research interests include glaucoma, neuro-ophthalmology, paediatric ophthalmology, and cataracts. She has authored over 80 scientific papers and edited two IntechOpen books. Dr. Ferreri is a member of several professional organizations, including the American Academy of Ophthalmology (AAO), the Italian Society of Ophthalmology (S.O.I.-A.M.O.I.), and the Italian Glaucoma Society (S.I.G.L.A.).

Contents

Preface IX

Chapter 1 1
Macular Corneal Dystrophy: Past, Present, and Future
by Aparajita Baruah, Sonjukta Borborah and Surya Prakash Goud Ponnam

Chapter 2 19
Promising New Options for Treating Microbial Keratitis
by Faisal Aljassar and Maryam Alsamhan

Chapter 3 35
Retinal Organoids: Advances in Generation, Development, and Applications – From Stem Cells to Disease Modeling and Regenerative Medicine
by Reyhaneh Sadat Mousavi, Fatemeh Naghshnejad, Fereshteh Karamali and Leila Satarian

Chapter 4 57
X-Linked Retinitis Pigmentosa Gene Therapy: Preclinical Aspects
by Vahid Mansouri and Maryam Bemanalizadeh

Chapter 5 85
Newer Medical Management Options in Glaucoma
by Sangeetha Sreenivasa Pai

Chapter 6 99
Exosomes and Exosome-Derived miRNAs: Current Knowledge and Future Aspects
by Ke Mao

Chapter 7 115
Indications and Surgical Treatments for Inherited Retinal Dystrophies
by Pamela Ríos and Cristina Irigoyen

Chapter 8 135
Penetrating Keratoplasty as an Inevitable Technique of Keratoplasty: Indications, Surgical Technique, and Outcomes
by Mathew Shemiakin and Gulzhiyan Arzhimatova

Chapter 9 153
Efficacy and Safety Analysis of 0.01% and 0.05% Atropine Combined with OK Lens in Children with Progressive Myopia
by Duo Xu, Yunyun Wang, Ling Ai, Benchu Feng, Zhilong Yang and Fuliang Li

Preface

The human eye is our primary interface with the external world. Over the past two decades, ophthalmology has evolved from a field limited by palliative care into a leader in precision medicine, regenerative therapies, and minimally invasive technologies. This volume, *Diseases of the Eye – Novel Investigations and Treatments*, captures this transformation by synthesizing cutting-edge science, clinical innovation, and patient-centered approaches across major ocular diseases.

Globally, the most common eye conditions include age-related macular degeneration (AMD), diabetic retinopathy (DR), glaucoma, cataracts, and dry eye disease. AMD affects over 190 million people and is the leading cause of irreversible central vision loss in older adults in developed nations. DR threatens vision in nearly one-third of people with diabetes. Glaucoma silently damages the optic nerve in more than 80 million individuals, half undiagnosed, while cataracts remain the top cause of blindness in low- and middle-income countries despite being surgically treatable. Dry eye disease, now recognized as a chronic, multifactorial disorder affecting up to 30% of adults, significantly impairs daily life.

Since the early 2000s, treatment paradigms have undergone a dramatic shift. Anti-VEGF therapies (e.g., ranibizumab, aflibercept, brolucizumab) revolutionized care for neovascular AMD and diabetic macular edema, halting progression and often restoring vision, redefining outcomes for millions. Glaucoma management has moved beyond topical medications, often limited by poor adherence and inconsistent IOP control, toward proactive strategies like minimally invasive glaucoma surgery (MIGS), first-line selective laser trabeculoplasty (SLT), and sustained-release drug delivery systems, enabling safer, earlier intervention and better long-term results.

Cataract surgery has become increasingly precise and personalized, with the assistance of femtosecond lasers and advanced intraocular lenses (e.g., trifocal, toric, extended depth-of-focus) that correct both cataracts and refractive errors, often eliminating the need for glasses. In dry eye disease, the recognition of inflammation as central to the pathogenesis has spurred the development of targeted treatments, including cyclosporine, lifitegrast, and autologous serum tears. Improved diagnostics, including meibography, tear osmolarity, and biomarker assays, support earlier detection. Meanwhile, thermal pulsation and intense pulsed light offer durable relief for meibomian gland dysfunction.

Emerging frontiers are equally promising: gene therapy has restored vision in inherited retinal dystrophies like Leber congenital amaurosis; stem cell-derived retinal pigment epithelium transplants show potential for geographic atrophy in AMD; artificial intelligence enhances screening for DR and glaucoma; and wearable biosensors enable continuous IOP monitoring for personalized management.

Collectively, these advances have repositioned ophthalmology as a proactive, predictive, and preventive specialty. Patients are no longer passive recipients of care but active participants in preserving, and sometimes regaining, functional vision. This progress demands continuous learning and adaptability from all eye care professionals.

This book is intended for a diverse yet discerning readership. Medical students will find a compelling introduction to the scientific and clinical foundations of modern ophthalmology that extends beyond conventional textbook summaries. Residents and fellows will benefit from concise, evidence-based updates on emerging diagnostics and therapeutics, bridging the gap between academic training and clinical practice. Practicing clinicians and surgeons will gain practical insights into integrating novel technologies, from MIGS devices to AI-enhanced imaging, into their workflows while navigating evolving regulatory and reimbursement frameworks. Researchers and biomedical engineers will find fertile ground for interdisciplinary collaboration, as chapters highlight unmet clinical needs, ongoing trials, and translational opportunities at the intersection of biology, engineering, and data science. Finally, policymakers, industry stakeholders, and educators will appreciate the balanced discussion of cost-effectiveness, accessibility, and ethical considerations that accompany rapid innovation.

Diseases of the Eye – Novel Investigations and Treatments is not merely a catalogue of new therapies and devices; it contextualizes these advancements within the lived experiences of patients and the evolving ethos of ophthalmic care. Each chapter, authored by leading experts, reflects technical excellence and a profound commitment to ophthalmology, where scientific progress serves the goal of preserving dignity, autonomy and human connection through vision.

This work would not have been possible without the exceptional dedication of our contributors. To each author and co-author: thank you for your scholarly rigour, clinical insight, and unwavering commitment to advancing the field. Your ability to distil complex concepts into accessible, actionable knowledge forms the cornerstone of this volume.

I also express my sincere gratitude to the editorial team at IntechOpen. Your professionalism, patience, and steadfast support throughout the planning, writing, and production phases were invaluable. Your commitment to open scientific exchange has played a pivotal role in bringing this project to fruition.

Felicia M. Ferreri
BIOMORF Department,
Messina, Italy

Chapter 1

Macular Corneal Dystrophy: Past, Present, and Future

Aparajita Baruah, Sonjukta Borborah and Surya Prakash Goud Ponnam

Abstract

Macular corneal dystrophy (MCD) is an autosomal recessive disorder of the human eye. It is characterized by gradual progress of the corneal opacities, resulting in loss of vision. Multiple studies from different ethnicities have identified at least 170 pathogenic mutations in the carbohydrate 6-sulfotransferase (*CHST6*) gene in MCD patients. More than 70% of these mutations have been observed in exon 3 of the *CHST6* gene. There is currently no medication to treat MCD, and surgery is the only available option. Clustered Regularly Interspaced Short Palindromic Repeats (CRISPR)/CRISPR-associated enzyme 9 (Cas9) is one of the most modern genome editing technologies that can be employed for precise genetic manipulations in different organisms across species. It consists of a Cas9 endonuclease protein that can be directed to cleave a target DNA sequence using a specifically designed guide RNA (gRNA). Further, advancements in CRISPR-Cas9-based genome editing technologies have aided in the emergence of novel therapeutic approaches for treating various human genetic disorders including ophthalmic diseases/disorders. In the proposed book chapter, we aim to focus on the various aspects of MCD, including the prevalence, molecular pathophysiology, genetics, available treatment options, CRISPR-Cas9, future therapeutic options using CRISPR-Cas technology, etc.

Keywords: genome editing, CRISPR-Cas9, macular corneal dystrophy, *CHST6*, cornea

1. Introduction

1.1 Macular corneal dystrophy (MCD)

Macular corneal dystrophy (MCD, OMIM #217800) is a human autosomal recessive disease/disorder that causes progressive corneal opacities resulting in bilateral vision loss. Besides a decrease in vision, the other clinical symptoms include pain and irritation in the eyes, photophobia, and a reduction in sensitivity of the cornea [1, 2]. The clinical signs and symptoms usually develop between the first and third decade of life, and the mean age of presentation is reported to be around 27 years [2, 3].

The carbohydrate-6-sulfotransferase (*CHST6*) gene (Ensembl ID: ENSG00000183196) has been reported to be associated with MCD. *CHST6* is located on chromosome 16q22 and has three exons. There are four available transcripts for the *CHST6* gene, out of which only two codes for the functional protein: corneal N-acetylglucosamine 6-0-sulfotransferase (c-GlcNAc6ST) (www.ensembl.org). The largest transcript (Ensemble ID: ENST00000332272.9) is approximately 8370 bp in length with 395 amino acids and has an approximate molecular weight of 44 kDa [4].

The function of the c-GlcNAc6ST protein is to transfer a sulfate group to the 6th position of the GlcNAc residues and participate in the keratan sulfate (KS) proteoglycan biosynthesis in the cornea [5]. KS preserves the size and structure of the cornea and maintains corneal hydration and transparency [6].

Depending on the presence or absence of keratan sulfate (KS) in the patient's serum and/or corneal tissues, MCD has been classified into three classes, and they are as follows:

a. MCD type I: No detectable keratan sulfate (KS) in the serum or cornea. Unsulfated keratan is present in the corneal endothelium, epithelium, and stroma.

b. MCD type IA: Absence of keratan sulfate in the serum, although KS is present in the stroma.

c. MCD type II: KS is present in both the cornea and serum. However, these MCD variants are clinically indistinguishable from each other [7].

2. Epidemiology

Macular corneal dystrophy is a type of corneal dystrophies. It comprises of around 10–75% of all the corneal dystrophies that require corneal grafting [8]. MCD has been reported from different populations across the globe that includes India [9, 10], Iceland [11], USA [12], Korea [13], Saudi Arabia [14], South Africa [15], Turkey [16], Iran [17], etc. Higher prevalence rates of MCD have been reported in Iceland, Saudi Arabia, and India [11, 14, 18]. The rates of prevalence of MCD have also been reported to be higher in communities with higher rates of consanguineous marriages [19].

The occurrence of MCD in the USA is 0.3 per 2,50,000 people [2]. Jonasson et al. reported that MCD was responsible for almost one-third of corneal grafts in the Icelandic population [11]. Two independent studies by Alzuhairy et al. and al Faran identified MCD as the most dominant form of corneal dystrophy in the Saudi Arabian population that required corneal transplantation [3, 14].

Multiple independent studies have been reported from India on the demographic, clinical, and molecular aspects of MCD. At least five studies were reported from Southern India, which included four from L. V. Prasad Eye Institute, Hyderabad, Telangana [10, 18, 20, 21] and one from Aravind Eye Hospital, Madurai, Tamil Nadu [9]. A study on MCD was also performed on patients reporting to AIIMS, New Delhi, an institute from Northern India [22]. The results from these studies have concluded that MCD is the second most common corneal dystrophy, with a prevalence rate of 29.3% [18, 21]. MCD type I was found to be the most common immunophenotype, followed by MCD type IA and type II [20]. Paliwal and co-workers reported that not all the individuals affected with MCD show mutations in the *CHST6* gene, indicating that other factors may also be responsible for the occurrence of MCD [22].

3. Pathogenesis

The most common symptoms associated with MCD include photophobia and gradual loss of vision in both eyes [2]. Approximately 170 mutations have been reported to be associated with the carbohydrate-6-sulfotransferase (*CHST6*) gene in different ethnicities across the globe (listed in **Table 1**). Due to the mutation in the *CHST6* gene, there is an

Phenotype	Codon change	Amino acid change	Population
Macular corneal dystrophy type I	ATG-TTG	M1L	North American
	CTC-CCC	L15P	French
	CAG-TAG	**Q18X**	**South Indian**
	CTC-CGC	**L22R**	**South Indian**
	CCC-TCC	P31S	British
	CAT-TAT	**H42Y**	**South Indian**
	CTG-CCG	L46P	North American
	CGC-CTC	**R50L**	**South Indian**
	TCG-TAG	S51X	Chinese
	TCG-TTG	S51L	Vietnamese
	GGC-GAC	**G52D**	**South Indian**
	TCG-TTG	**S53L**	**South Indian**
	TCC-TTC	**S54F**	**South Indian**
	CAA-TAA	Q58X	French
	CTC-CCC	L59P	Vietnamese
	AAC-ACC	N61T	French
	CAC-CAG	H63Q	North American
	GTC-CTC	V66L	Vietnamese
	TAC-CAC	Y68H	French
	ATG-AAG	M70K	French
	CCC-TCC	P72S	British
	GCG-ACG	**A73T**	**South Indian**
	GCG-CCG	A73P	North American
	GTG-ATG	V76M	Vietnamese
	TGG-TGA	W77X	North American
	CAG-TAG	Q82X	French
	GTG-CTG	V92L	North American
	CGC-CAC	**R93H**	**South Indian**
	CGC-CCC	**R97P**	**South Indian**
	TGC-GGC	C102G	French
	TGC-TAC	**C102Y**	**South Indian**
	ATG-GTG	M104V	North American

Phenotype	Codon change	Amino acid change	Population
	TTT-TCT	F107S	British
	TAT-TGT	Y110C	North American
	CGC-TGC	R114C	North American
	TTC-TCC	**F121S**	**South Indian**
	TTC-TTG	**F121L**	**South Indian**
	TGG-TGA	**W123X**	**South Indian**
	CGT-TGT	**R127C**	**South Indian**
	GCA-GTA	A128V	Icelandic
	TCG-CCG	S131P	French
	TCG-TTG	S131L	North American
	CGA-TGA	R140X	British
	CTG-CCG	L152P	French
	TGC-TGA	**C153X**	**South Indian**
	TGC-TGG	**C165W**	**South Indian**
	CGC-CCC	R166P	Icelandic
	TCC-TTC	**S167F**	**South Indian**
	AAG-AGG	K174R	North American
	GTG-ATG	V176M	Turkish
	CGC-CAC	R177H	Japanese
	CGC-GGC	R177G	North American
	CGC-TGC	R177C	North American
	TTC-TGC	**F178C**	**South Indian**
	CTC-CCC	**L193P**	**South Indian**
	GTG-GAG	V198E	Italian
	CTG-CGG	L200R	British
	CGC-AGC	**R202S**	**South Indian**
	GAC-AAC	D203N	North American
	GAC-GAA	D203E	North American
	CCG-CAG	P204Q	Japanese
	CCG-CGG	**P204R**	**South Indian**
	CCG-TCG	P204S	Turkish
	CGG-CAG	**R205Q**	**South Indian**
	CGG-CTG	R205L	Japanese
	GCC-ACC	**A206T**	**South Indian**
	GCC-GTC	A206V	British
	TCC-TTC	**S210F**	**South Indian**
	CGG-CAG	R211Q	Vietnamese
	CGG-TGG	R211W	North American

Phenotype	Codon change	Amino acid change	Population
	GCT-ACT	A217T	North American
	GAC-GAG	**D221E**	**South Indian**
	GAC-TAC	**D221Y**	**South Indian**
	TGG-TGA	W232X	Vietnamese
	TGC-TGG	C246W	North American
	AGC-AGG	S248R	North American
	CAC-CCC	**H249P**	**South Indian**
	TAC-TGC	Y268C	Vietnamese
	CGC-AGC	**R272S**	**South Indian**
	CGC-CAC	R272H	North American
	GGA-TGA	**G309X**	**South Indian**
	CAG-TAG	Q331X	North American
	CGC-TGC	**R334C**	**South Indian**
	GAA-TAA	**E347X**	**South Indian**
	TGC-TAC	C349Y	North American
	TGC-TGG	C349W	North American
	TAC-GAC	Y358D	British
Macular corneal dystrophy type II	CGC-TGC	R50C	North American
	TTC-TCC	F55S	Turkish
	TGG-TGC	W77C	North American
	CGC-AGC	R93S	North American
	CAG-CCG	Q122P	North American
	CCG-CGG	P186R	North American
	CTG-CCG	L276P	North American
	GTC-CTC	V329L	Icelandic

Table 1.
The list of a few mutations in the CHST6 gene associated with the types of MCD across the globe (www.hgmd.org) and from India [highlighted in bold].

abnormal deposition of glycosaminoglycan in the corneal stroma, the Descemet membrane, keratocytes, and the endothelium. This ultimately leads to the occurrence of a hazy stroma and the loss of corneal transparency [23]. Two independent studies (Klintworth et al. 1986 and Thonar et al. 1986) have reported that patients with MCD type I and IA do not have detectable keratan sulfate in the serum; however, normal levels of keratan sulfate can be observed in the serum of patients with MCD type II [24, 25].

4. Genetics

Corneal dystrophies represent a group of genetic disorders that are usually bilateral and affect corneal transparency and vision [26]. The International

Committee for Classification of Corneal Dystrophies (IC3D) has categorized corneal dystrophies (CDs) into four different classes: (a) Epithelial and subepithelial CDs; (b) Epithelial-stromal TGFBI CDs; (c) stromal CDs; and (d) endothelial CDs [27].

In 1890, Groenouw reported two cases of corneal dystrophy, which he believed to be two different variations of the same disease. Later, these corneal dystrophies were recognized as macular corneal dystrophy (MCD) and granular corneal dystrophy (GCD) [28]. Molecular characterization of corneal dystrophies revealed both genetic heterogeneities, with different genes (*KRT3* and *KRT12*) being responsible for the occurrence of a single disease phenotype (Meesmann Corneal Dystrophy), and phenotypic heterogeneity, that is, a single gene (*TGFBI*) being associated with different disease phenotypes (Thiel-Behnke dystrophy, Reis-Bücklers corneal dystrophy, granular corneal dystrophy, and lattice corneal dystrophy) [29].

Most of the corneal dystrophies exhibit an autosomal dominant pattern of inheritance. However, even autosomal recessive modes of inheritance do exist in a few forms of the disease, including macular corneal dystrophy (MCD) and congenital hereditary corneal dystrophy (CHED) [30, 31].

Vance et al. reported the linkage of human chromosome number 16 to both MCD type I and type II in populations from the United States and Iceland [32]. Akama et al. have reported the association of the Carbohydrate sulfotransferase gene (*CHST6*) with type I MCD [33]. Most of the patients with MCD are reported to have homozygous variations in the *CHST6* gene [5, 19]. Abbruzzese C and co-workers have observed that MCD type I occurs mostly due to missense mutations in the coding region of the *CHST6* gene; however, large deletion and replacement in the upstream region of *CHST6* were associated with type II MCD [6]. However, there was no correlation observed between the genotypes and phenotypes of the patients with MCD [20].

Of all the mutations reported in *CHST6* globally, more than 50% have been reported from India [34], and this is a matter of great concern. More than a hundred of the missense mutations (approximately 70% of the total mutations) are reported in the third exon of the *CHST6* gene (www.hgmd.org). A few pathogenic mutations associated with the type of MCD, the codon change, and the corresponding amino acid change in different populations across the globe are listed in **Table 1**.

5. Current treatment modalities

Penetrating keratoplasty (PKP) and Deep anterior lamellar keratoplasty (DALK) are few of the surgical techniques that have been used in the treatment of MCD [35, 36]. DALK is proven to be an efficient surgical procedure that reduces the chances of endothelial damage and endothelial rejection post-treatment and almost 75% of the restoration of vision in MCD patients [36, 37]. However, AlAraj and co-workers have reported that there was no significant difference in the restoration of vision in patients who underwent either DALK or PKP surgery [38]. There are several challenges associated with these surgeries including recurrence, rejection of the endothelium, and loss of endothelial cells [39].

6. Gene therapy

6.1 Clustered regularly interspaced short palindromic repeats (CRISPR)-CRISPR-associated protein 9 (Cas9)

The genome editing technologies have evolved with time, starting with the meganucleases, zinc-finger nucleases (ZFNs), transcription activator-like effector nucleases (TALENs), and the latest being the CRISPR-Cas technology [40].

Clustered Regularly Interspaced Short Palindromic Repeats (CRISPR) is a prokaryotic acquired immune response mechanism developed for protection against pathogens such as viruses. The CRISPR locus comprises an array of spacers interspaced with short repetitive sequences and the Cas gene. CRISPR utilizes guide RNA sequences to direct the Cas proteins toward the target genomic locations [41].

Based on the Cas protein variant, there are two different classes of the CRISPR-Cas system that can further be divided into six different types (I–VI). Class 1 systems (types I, III, and IV) consist of multiple Cas effector proteins, while Class 2 systems (types II, V, and VI) consist of a single Cas effector protein. Types I, II, IV, and V target DNA; type III targets both DNA and RNA; while type VI specifically targets RNA [42].

6.2 Mechanism of action of CRISPR-Cas9

The CRISPR-Cas9 system consists of a crRNA that forms the guide RNA (gRNA), a transactivating crRNA (tracrRNA) that facilitates the maturation of the crRNA, and a Cas9 endonuclease [43]. The guide RNA (gRNA) directs the Cas9 to any target DNA sequence adjacent to a Protospacer Adjacent Motif (PAM) [44]. The PAM site interacts with Arg1333 and Arg1335 amino acids of the Cas9 in order to form a phosphate lock loop around the target site [45]. Structural analysis of the sgRNA-Cas9 complex and target DNA revealed the formation of an RNA-DNA hybrid (R-loop) [46]. Cas9 consists of two different domains: the HNH domain, which cleaves the DNA strand complementary to the spacer, while the RuvC domain cleaves the non-complementary strand [47].

6.3 Challenges with CRISPR-Cas and possible solutions

Although the RNA-guided Cas9 is an efficient genome editing tool, it has been reported to show limitations like "off-target" activity, not so efficient Cas9, immunogenicity, polymorphisms and inefficient delivery of the Cas9 into the target sites [48, 49].

Multiple approaches have been described by researchers to enhance the efficiency of CRISPR-Cas9, and these include improving the designing and efficiency of the gRNA to guide the cas9 protein at the desired site, enhancing the efficiency of Cas9 by introducing various modifications into the Cas protein, and also designing efficient methods of Cas9 delivery into the cells.

6.3.1 Efficient designing of gRNA

To design efficient gRNAs, few studies have reported the optimal length of gRNAs to be between 15 to 20 nucleotides [50, 51]. Various bioinformatics tools and software, such as CHOPCHOP, CRISPOR etc., have been developed that predict the efficiency and reduces the off-target modifications [52, 53].

6.3.2 Modifications of the Cas9 protein

To achieve greater on-target and reduced off-target activity, multiple variants of the Cas9 protein have been developed, including Cas9 nickases (nCas9), catalytically dead Cas9 (dCas9) nucleases, high-fidelity CRISPR-Cas9 (SpCas9-HF1), and enhanced specificity Cas9 (eSpCas9) [54]. The dCas9 and nCas9 have no nuclease activity, but they retain the DNA targeting [55, 56].

The immediate requirement of PAM (protospacer-adjacent motif) sequence near the DNA target site poses a limitation on the number of editable sequences. To mitigate this constraint, Cas9 variants with relaxed PAM requirements and near-PAMless variants are developed like SpG-Cas9 (SpG), SpRY-Cas9 (SpRY), SpCas9-NG, etc. [57, 58]. SuperFi-Cas9, an increased-fidelity nuclease (IFN), when combined with cytosine base editors (CBE) and adenine base editors (ABE), has been proven to show highly efficient DNA editing [59].

A recent addition to the list is a Cas9 isolated from *Francisella novicida* (FnCas9). This is reported to have high precision with a negligible affinity for mismatched substrates. However, its low cellular targeting efficiency limits its therapeutic use [60]. The latest version of the Cas9 reported is enhanced (en) FnCas9, with single mismatch specificity, for improved gene editing. There are five variants of the enFnCas9: en1, en15, en31, en34, and en40, which have relaxed PAM requirements and demonstrated enhanced on-target activity when compared to regular FnCas9 [61].

6.3.3 Efficient delivery systems

Multiple strategies have been developed for efficient delivery of the Cas9 into cells of choice, some of which include electroporation, viral vector-mediated transfer, and nanoparticles.

Kim et al. have reported the delivery of Cas9-sgRNA complex into human cells through electroporation, which was difficult to transfect, including fibroblasts and pluripotent stem cells [62]. Yang et al. employed a dual AAV (Adeno-associated virus) system (one containing the gRNA and the template DNA, and the other containing the Cas9 protein) for the successful correction of metabolic liver disease in mice [63]. Stephens et al. have reported CRISPR/Cas9 delivery *via* AdVs (Adenoviruses) to successfully knock in human alpha-1-antitrypsin into the *ROSA26* gene in murine livers [64]. Finn and co-workers reported successful *in vivo* delivery of the Cas9 mRNA and sgRNA, which reduced the TTR protein production level by approximately 97% in a mouse model [65]. Zhao et al. have reported AAV-mediated CRISPR/Cas9 correction of the mutated *LDLR* gene and reduced expression of atherosclerosis phenotypes in a mouse model [66]. Cationic polymers like polyethyleneimine and chitosan have been used to deliver nucleic acids, plasmid DNA, and mRNA into human cell lines [67].

6.4 Therapeutic applications of CRISPR-Cas

Due to the versatile nature of the CRISPR/Cas and the possibility to modify the guide RNA sequence to edit a diverse array of genes, this new generation technology is employed to target pathogenic DNA variations, offering potential disease treatment opportunities both *in vivo* and *in vitro* [68, 69]. A few of the studies are discussed here.

6.4.1 In vitro *studies*

Smith et al. used CRISPR-Cas9 to rectify mutations in the JAK2 and *AAT* genes in patient-derived iPSCs [70]. Maurya et al. and Moses et al. demonstrated the correction of mutations in tumor suppressor genes like *PKC* and *PTEN* using CRISPR-Cas9 [71, 72]. Two independent studies by Firth et al. and Marangi et al. have reported significant correction of deletion mutation in the *CFTR* gene in iPSCs derived from cystic fibrosis patients using the CRISPR-Cas9 system [73, 74]. Shin et al. and Monteys et al. used CRISPR-Cas9 in fibroblast cells of patients with Huntington's disease to modify the pathogenic CAG repeats within the *HTT* gene [75, 76]. Scharenberg et al. developed CRISPR-mediated cell therapy for Gaucher disease by knocking in glucocerebrosidase (GCase) into the *CCR5* safe-harbor locus in hematopoietic stem cells, restoring GCase expression in monocyte-macrophage lineage cells [77]. Maxwell et al. corrected *WFS1* gene mutations in induced pluripotent stem cells (iPSCs) from patients with Wolfram syndrome and showed an increase in insulin secretion in a diabetic mouse model [78]. Christie and co-workers incorporated CRISPR-Cas9 to edit mutations in the *TGFBI* gene, which was capable of differentiating between the two alleles of the target gene [79]. Frangoul and group reported successful gene therapy for sickle cell and β-thalassemia diseases by editing the *BCL11A* gene to restore γ-globin expression [80].

6.4.2 In vivo *studies*

Cwerman-Thibault et al. introduced a recombinant adeno-associated viral vector containing NADH dehydrogenase subunit 4 (ND4) into a rat model of Leber hereditary optic neuropathy (LHON), demonstrating prevention of retinal ganglion cell degeneration [81]. Courtney et al. had demonstrated that by editing the mutant *KRT12* gene in a mouse mode, Meesmann's epithelial corneal dystrophy (MECD) could be treated through CRISPR/Cas9-based therapeutics [82]. Li et al. observed that sub-retinal injection of sgRNA-Cas9 constructs into mice with Retinitis pigmentosa resulted in reduced expression of the mutant gene and slowing down photoreceptor cell degeneration [83]. A report by Amoasii et al. has demonstrated the correction of mutations in the 51st exon of the Dystrophin gene in a dog model using CRISPR-Cas9, which ultimately restored normal protein expression [84]. Similarly, Ekman et al. abolished the expression of the mutant *HTT* gene in mice model that resulted in a significant decrease in neuronal inclusions, improved lifespan, and motor function [85]. In a clinical trial by Gilmore et al., intravenous infusion of lipid nanoparticles (LNPs) containing SpCas9 and sgRNA targeting the mutated Transthyretin (*TTR*) gene showed more than 95% reduction in the level of misfolded TTR protein in the patient's serum [86].

7. dsDNA repair mechanism

In eukaryotes, CRISPR-Cas9-induced double-strand breaks (DSBs) are repaired *via* three main repair pathways: homologous recombination (HR), non-homologous end joining (NHEJ), and microhomology-mediated end joining (MMEJ) [87]. HR is active during the S and G2 phases of the cell cycle and is generally error-free as it uses a homologous DNA sequence as a template [88]. NHEJ, on the other hand, functions throughout the cell cycle and is the primary mechanism of DSB repair [89]. MMEJ, an alternative NHEJ process, is active during the G1 and early S phases and utilizes short homologous sequences near the DSB site for repair. The NHEJ is an error-prone mechanism and often involves random insertions and deletions (INDELs) at the cut site. This may result in frameshift mutations, introducing a premature stop codon, or creating a non-functional protein [90].

Therefore, these pathways may be avoided when genome editing is planned for. It has been reported that downregulation of the few genes associated with the NHEJ pathway increases the efficiency of HR-mediated genome editing in mammalian cell lines. Maruyama et al. reported that HR-mediated DSB repair efficiency increased by 19-fold upon the expression of DNA ligase IV, a key factor of the NHEJ pathway, was blocked using an inhibitor, Scr7 [91]. Li and co-workers reported that siRNA-mediated downregulation of the two major proteins (Ku70 and Ku80) of the NHEJ pathway resulted in the enhancement of HDR frequency in pig fetal fibroblast cells [92]. A recent study by Wang and co-workers proved the CRISPR/Cas9-mediated knockout of the *LIG4* gene, involved in NHEJ, increases the efficiency of site-specific integration in Chinese hamster ovary cell line [93].

8. Conclusion

Macular corneal dystrophy is an autosomal recessive disorder of human that is characterized by the abnormality in the biosynthesis of proteoglycan. With more than 50% of the mutations in the *CHST6* gene in the third exon, we believe that the third exon of the *CHST6* gene could be the potential region of interest for genome editing. Gene therapy for MCD may be challenging considering the huge number of mutations spread across the *CHST6* gene and hardly any recurrent mutation among MCD patients. However, a part of the exon of the *CHST6* gene with maximum mutations can be targeted using gene therapy, including CRISPR-Cas9 technology.

In vitro experiments can be performed to modify a fragment of the third exon of the *CHST6* gene *via* the CRISPR/Cas system using Cas9 or other high-efficiency nucleases and by supplying a functional donor template in human cell lines as a proof of concept. In order to promote the HR pathway and increase the editing efficiency, we may knock down/downregulate a few proteins involved in the NHEJ pathway and bias the cells toward MMEJ/HR pathways in immortalized human corneal keratinocytes (IHCK) and/or induced pluripotent stem cells (iPSCs) derived from MCD patients.

Further, *in vivo* assessment can be performed by editing the pathogenic mutations in the *CHST6* gene in disease animal models and testing for the restoration of vision using CRISPR-Cas9-based technology. This may be a novel potential therapeutic option for the treatment of one of the highly prevalent forms of hereditary corneal dystrophy, MCD.

Acknowledgements

Ms. Aparajita Baruah acknowledges financial support in the form of CSIR-JRF and SRF fellowship, Govt. of India. Ms. Sonjukta Borborah acknowledges the financial support received in the form of an Institutional fellowship for research scholars from Tezpur University. The authors acknowledge the infrastructural support from Tezpur University.

Conflict of interest

The authors declare no conflict of interest.

Author details

Aparajita Baruah, Sonjukta Borborah and Surya Prakash Goud Ponnam*
Department of Molecular Biology and Biotechnology, School of Sciences, Tezpur University, Sonitpur, Assam, India

*Address all correspondence to: surya_p@tezu.ac.in

References

[1] Klintworth GK. Corneal dystrophies. Orphanet Journal of Rare Diseases. 2009; **4**:7. DOI: 10.1186/1750-1172-4-723

[2] Aggarwal S, Peck T, Golen J, et al. Macular corneal dystrophy: A review. Survey of Ophthalmology. 2018;**63**(5): 609-617. DOI: 10.1016/j.survophthal.2018.03.004

[3] Alzuhairy S, Alkatan HM, Al-Rajhi AA. Prevalence and histopathological characteristics of corneal stromal dystrophies in Saudi Arabia. Middle East African Journal of Ophthalmology. 2015; **22**(2):179-185. DOI: 10.4103/0974-9233.151975

[4] Zhang J, Wu D, Li Y, et al. A comprehensive evaluation of 181 reported CHST6 variants in patients with macular corneal dystrophy. Aging (Albany NY). 2019;**11**(3):1019-1029. DOI: 10.18632/aging.101807

[5] Liu NP, Smith CF, Bowling BL, et al. Macular corneal dystrophy types I and II are caused by distinct mutations in the CHST6 gene in Iceland. Molecular Vision. 2006;**12**:1148-1152

[6] Abbruzzese C, Kuhn U, Molina F, et al. Novel mutations in the CHST6 gene causing macular corneal dystrophy. Clinical Genetics. 2004;**65**(2):120-125. DOI: 10.1111/j.0009-9163.2004.00191.x

[7] Jonasson F, Oshima E, Thonar EJ, et al. Macular corneal dystrophy in Iceland. A clinical, genealogic, and immunohistochemical study of 28 patients. Ophthalmology. 1996;**103**(7): 1111-1117. DOI: 10.1016/s0161-6420(96)30559-9

[8] El-Ashry MF, Abd El-Aziz MM, Wilkins S, et al. Identification of novel mutations in the carbohydrate sulfotransferase gene (CHST6) causing macular corneal dystrophy. Investigative Ophthalmology & Visual Science. 2002; **43**(2):377-382

[9] Warren JF, Aldave AJ, Srinivasan M, et al. Novel mutations in the CHST6 gene associated with macular corneal dystrophy in southern India. Archives of Ophthalmology. 2003;**121**(11): 1608-1612. DOI: 10.1001/archopht.121.11.1608

[10] Sultana A, Sridhar MS, Jagannathan A, et al. Novel mutations of the carbohydrate sulfotransferase-6 (CHST6) gene causing macular corneal dystrophy in India. Molecular Vision. 2003;**9**:730-734

[11] Jonasson F, Johannsson JH, Garner A, et al. Macular corneal dystrophy in Iceland. Eye (London, England). 1989;**3**(Pt 4):446-454. DOI: 10.1038/eye.1989.66

[12] Aldave AJ, Yellore VS, Thonar EJ, et al. Novel mutations in the carbohydrate sulfotransferase gene (CHST6) in American patients with macular corneal dystrophy. American Journal of Ophthalmology. 2004;**137**(3): 465-473. DOI: 10.1016/j.ajo.2003.09.036

[13] Park SH, Ahn YJ, Chae H, et al. Molecular analysis of the CHST6 gene in Korean patients with macular corneal dystrophy: Identification of three novel mutations. Molecular Vision. 2015;**21**: 1201-1209

[14] al Faran MF, Tabbara KF. Corneal dystrophies among patients undergoing keratoplasty in Saudi Arabia. Cornea. 1991;**10**(1):13-16

[15] Carstens N, Williams S, Goolam S, et al. Novel mutation in the CHST6 gene

causes macular corneal dystrophy in a black South African family. BMC Medical Genetics. 2016;**17**(1):47. DOI: 10.1186/s12881-016-0308-0

[16] Yaylacioglu Tuncay F, Kayman Kurekci G, Guntekin Ergun S, et al. Genetic analysis of CHST6 and TGFBI in Turkish patients with corneal dystrophies: Five novel variations in CHST6. Molecular Vision. 2016;**22**: 1267-1279

[17] Birgani SA, Salehi Z, Houshmand M, et al. Novel mutations of CHST6 in Iranian patients with macular corneal dystrophy. Molecular Vision. 2009;**15**: 373-377

[18] Pandrowala H, Bansal A, Vemuganti GK, et al. Frequency, distribution, and outcome of keratoplasty for corneal dystrophies at a tertiary eye care center in South India. Cornea. 2004;**23**(6):541-546. DOI: 10.1097/01.ico.0000126324.58884.b9

[19] Singh S, Das S, Kannabiran C, et al. Macular corneal dystrophy: An updated review. Current Eye Research. 2021; **46**(6):765-770. DOI: 10.1080/02713683.2020.1849727

[20] Sultana A, Klintworth GK, Thonar EJ, et al. Immunophenotypes of macular corneal dystrophy in India and correlation with mutations in CHST6. Molecular Vision. 2009;**15**: 319-325

[21] Das AV, Chaurasia S. Clinical profile and demographic distribution of corneal dystrophies in India: A study of 4198 patients. Cornea. 2021;**40**(5):548-553. DOI: 10.1097/ICO.0000000000002450

[22] Paliwal P, Sharma A, Tandon R, et al. Molecular genetic analysis of macular corneal dystrophy patients from North India. Ophthalmic Research. 2012;**48**(1): 28-32. DOI: 10.1159/000334911

[23] Dudakova L, Palos M, Svobodova M, et al. Macular corneal dystrophy and associated corneal thinning. Eye (London, England). 2014;**28**(10): 1201-1205. DOI: 10.1038/eye.2014.164

[24] Klintworth GK, Meyer R, Dennis R, et al. Macular corneal dystrophy. Lack of keratan sulfate in serum and cornea. Ophthalmic Paediatrics and Genetics. 1986;**7**:139-143. DOI: 10.3109/13816818609004130

[25] Thonar EJ, Meyer RF, Dennis RF, et al. Absence of normal keratan sulfate in the blood of patients with macular corneal dystrophy. American Journal of Ophthalmology. 1986;**102**(5):561-569. DOI: 10.1016/0002-9394(86)90525-8

[26] Soh YQ, Kocaba V, Weiss JS, et al. Corneal dystrophies. Nature Reviews. Disease Primers. 2020;**6**(1):46. DOI: 10.1038/s41572-020-0178-9

[27] Weiss JS, Møller HU, Aldave AJ, et al. IC3D classification of corneal dystrophies–edition 2. Cornea. 2015; **34**(2):117-159. DOI: 10.1097/ICO.0000000000000307

[28] Groenouw A. Knoetchenfoermige Hornhauttruebungen (Noduli corneae). Arch Augenheilkd. 1890;**21**:281-289

[29] Weiss JS, Møller HU, Lisch W, et al. The IC3D classification of the corneal dystrophies. Cornea. 2008;**27**(Suppl 2): S1-S83. DOI: 10.1097/ICO.0b013e31817780fb

[30] Lisch W, Weiss JS. Clinical and genetic update of corneal dystrophies. Experimental Eye Research. 2019;**186**: 107715. DOI: 10.1016/j.exer.2019.107715. Epub 2019 Jul 10. Erratum in: Exp Eye

Res. 2020 Mar;192:107929. DOI: 10.1016/j.exer.2020.107929

[31] Sacchetti M, Macchi I, Tiezzi A, et al. Pathophysiology of corneal dystrophies: From cellular genetic alteration to clinical findings. Journal of Cellular Physiology. 2016;**231**(2):261-269. DOI: 10.1002/jcp.25082

[32] Vance JM, Jonasson F, Lennon F, et al. Linkage of a gene for macular corneal dystrophy to chromosome 16. American Journal of Human Genetics. 1996;**58**(4):757-762

[33] Akama T, Nishida K, Nakayama J, et al. Macular corneal dystrophy type I and type II are caused by distinct mutations in a new sulfotransferase gene. Nature Genetics. 2000;**26**:237-241

[34] Sultana A, Sridhar MS, Klintworth GK, et al. Allelic heterogeneity of the carbohydrate sulfotransferase-6 gene in patients with macular corneal dystrophy. Clinical Genetics. 2005;**68**(5):454-460. DOI: 10.1111/j.1399-0004.2005.00517.x

[35] Al-Swailem SA, Al-Rajhi AA, Wagoner MD. Penetrating keratoplasty for macular corneal dystrophy. Ophthalmology. 2005;**11**(2):220-224. DOI: 10.1016/j.ophtha.2004.08.01712

[36] Unal M, Arslan OS, Atalay E, et al. Deep anterior lamellar keratoplasty for the treatment of stromal corneal dystrophies. Cornea. 2013;**32**(3): 301-305. DOI: 10.1097/ICO.0b013e31825718ca

[37] Sogutlu Sari E, Kubaloglu A, Unal M, et al. Deep anterior lamellar keratoplasty versus penetrating keratoplasty for macular corneal dystrophy: A randomized trial. American Journal of Ophthalmology. 2013;**156**(2):267-274.e1. DOI: 10.1016/j.ajo.2013.03.007

[38] AlAraj A, AlAmeer A, Al-Swailem S. Medium-term clinical outcomes of deep anterior lamellar keratoplasty versus penetrating keratoplasty for macular corneal dystrophy. Clinical Ophthalmology. 2021;**23**(15):3139-3145. DOI: 10.2147/OPTH.S317971

[39] Marcon AS, Cohen EJ, Rapuano CJ, et al. Recurrence of corneal stromal dystrophies after penetrating keratoplasty. Cornea. 2003;**22**(1):19-21. DOI: 10.1097/00003226-200301000-00005

[40] Wang H, La Russa M, Qi LS. CRISPR/Cas9 in genome editing and beyond. Annual Review of Biochemistry. 2016;**85**:227-264. DOI: 10.1146/annurev-biochem-060815-014607

[41] Doudna JA, Charpentier E, Genome editing. The new frontier of genome engineering with CRISPR-Cas9. Science. 2014;**346**(6213):1258096. DOI: 10.1126/science.1258096

[42] Murjani K, Tripathi R, Singh V. An overview and potential of CRISPR-Cas systems for genome editing. Progress in Molecular Biology and Translational Science. 2024;**208**:1-17. DOI: 10.1016/bs.pmbts.2024.07.009

[43] Ran F, Hsu P, Wright J, et al. Genome engineering using the CRISPR-Cas9 system. Nature Protocols. 2013;**8**: 2281-2308. DOI: 10.1038/nprot.2013.143

[44] Park CS, Habib O, Lee Y, et al. Applications of CRISPR technologies to the development of gene and cell therapy. BMB Reports. 2024;**57**(1):2-11. DOI: 10.5483/BMBRep.2023-0221

[45] Kleinstiver BP, Prew MS, Tsai SQ, et al. Engineered CRISPR-Cas9 nucleases with altered PAM specificities. Nature. 2015;**523**(7561):481-485. DOI: 10.1038/nature14592

[46] Jiang F, Taylor DW, Chen JS, et al. Structures of a CRISPR-Cas9 R-loop complex primed for DNA cleavage. Science. 2016;**351**(6275):867-871. DOI: 10.1126/science.aad8282

[47] Kulishova LM, Vokhtantsev IP, Kim DV, et al. Mechanism of the CRISPR/Cas9 System Specificity in Genome Editing. Molekulârnaâ biologiâ. 2023;**57**(2):269-284. DOI: 10.31857/S0026898423020155

[48] Guo C, Ma X, Gao F, et al. Off-target effects in CRISPR/Cas9 gene editing. Frontiers in Bioengineering and Biotechnology. 2023;**11**:1143157. Published 2023 Mar 9. DOI: 10.3389/fbioe.2023.1143157

[49] Liu W, Li L, Jiang J, Wu M, et al. Applications and challenges of CRISPR-Cas gene editing to disease treatment in clinics. Precision Clinical Medicine. 2021;**4**(3):179-191. DOI: 10.1093/pcmedi/pbab014

[50] Hazafa A, Mumtaz M, Farooq MF, et al. CRISPR/Cas9: A powerful genome editing technique for the treatment of cancer cells with present challenges and future directions. Life Sciences. 2020;**15**(263):118525. DOI: 10.1016/j.lfs.2020.118525

[51] Lv J, Wu S, Wei R, et al. The length of guide RNA and target DNA heteroduplex effects on CRISPR/Cas9 mediated genome editing efficiency in porcine cells. Journal of Veterinary Science. 2019;**20**(3):e23

[52] Concordet J-P, Haeussler M. CRISPOR: Intuitive guide selection for CRISPR/Cas9 genome editing experiments and screens. Nucleic Acids Research. 2018;**46**(W1):W242-W245. DOI: 10.1093/nar/gky354

[53] Labun K, Montague TG, Gagnon JA, et al. CHOPCHOP v2: A web tool for the next generation of CRISPR genome engineering. Nucleic Acids Research. 2016;**44**(W1):W272-W276. DOI: 10.1093/nar/gkw398

[54] Chen F, Ding X, Feng Y, et al. Targeted activation of diverse CRISPR-Cas systems for mammalian genome editing via proximal CRISPR targeting. Nature Communications. 2017;**8**:14958. Published 2017 Apr 7. DOI: 10.1038/ncomms14958

[55] Lee J, Lim K, Kim A, et al. Prime editing with genuine Cas9 nickases minimizes unwanted indels. Nature Communications. 2023;**14**:1786. DOI: 10.1038/s41467-023-37507-8

[56] Cai R, Lv R, Shi X, et al. CRISPR/dCas9 tools: Epigenetic mechanism and application in gene transcriptional regulation. International Journal of Molecular Sciences. 2023;**24**(19):14865. DOI: 10.3390/ijms241914865

[57] Walton RT, Christie KA, Whittaker MN, et al. Unconstrained genome targeting with near-PAMless engineered CRISPR-Cas9 variants. Science. 2020;**368**(6488):290-296. DOI: 10.1126/science.aba8853

[58] Nishimasu H, Shi X, Ishiguro S, et al. Engineered CRISPR-Cas9 nuclease with expanded targeting space. Science. 2018;**361**(6408):1259-1262. DOI: 10.1126/science.aas9129

[59] Kulcsár PI, Tálas A, Ligeti Z, et al. SuperFi-Cas9 exhibits remarkable fidelity but severely reduced activity yet works effectively with ABE8e. Nature Communications. 2022;**13**(1):6858. DOI: 10.1038/s41467-022-34527-8

[60] Acharya S, Mishra A, Paul D, et al. *Francisella novicida* Cas9 interrogates

genomic DNA with very high specificity and can be used for mammalian genome editing. Proceedings of the National Academy of Sciences of the United States of America. 2019;**116**(42): 20959-20968. DOI: 10.1073/pnas.1818461116

[61] Acharya S, Ansari AH, Kumar Das P, et al. PAM-flexible engineered FnCas9 variants for robust and ultra-precise genome editing and diagnostics. Nature Communications. 2024;**15**:5471. DOI: 10.1038/s41467-024-49233-w

[62] Kim S, Kim D, Cho SW, et al. Highly efficient RNA-guided genome editing in human cells via delivery of purified Cas9 ribonucleoproteins. Genome Research. 2014;**24**(6):1012-1019. DOI: 10.1101/gr.171322.113

[63] Yang Y, Wang L, Bell P, et al. A dual AAV system enables the Cas9-mediated correction of a metabolic liver disease in newborn mice. Nature Biotechnology. 2016;**34**(3):334-338. DOI: 10.1038/nbt.3469

[64] Stephens CJ, Kashentseva E, Everett W, et al. Targeted in vivo knock-in of human alpha-1-antitrypsin cDNA using adenoviral delivery of CRISPR/Cas9. Gene Therapy. 2018;**25**(2):139-156. DOI: 10.1038/s41434-018-0003-1

[65] Finn JD, Smith AR, Patel MC, et al. A single administration of CRISPR/Cas9 lipid nanoparticles achieves robust and persistent *in vivo* Genome editing. Cell Reports. 2018;**22**(9):2227-2235. DOI: 10.1016/j.celrep.2018.02.014

[66] Zhao H, Li Y, He L, et al. *In vivo* AAV-CRISPR/Cas9-mediated gene editing ameliorates atherosclerosis in familial hypercholesterolemia. Circulation. 2020;**141**(1):67-79. DOI: 10.1161/CIRCULATIONAHA.119.042476

[67] Duan L, Ouyang K, Xu X, et al. Nanoparticle delivery of CRISPR/Cas9 for genome editing. Frontiers in Genetics. 2021;**12**:673286. DOI: 10.3389/fgene.2021.673286

[68] Jo DH, Song DW, Cho CS, et al. CRISPR-Cas9-mediated therapeutic editing of Rpe65 ameliorates the disease phenotypes in a mouse model of Leber congenital amaurosis. Science Advances. 2019;**5**(10):eaax1210. DOI: 10.1126/sciadv.aax1210

[69] Witz A, Dardare J, Francois A, et al. CRISPR/Cas9-mediated knock-in of BRCA1/2 mutations restores response to olaparib in pancreatic cancer cell lines. Scientific Reports. 2023;**13**(1):18741. DOI: 10.1038/s41598-023-45964-w

[70] Smith C, Abalde-Atristain L, He C, et al. Efficient and allele-specific genome editing of disease loci in human iPSCs. Molecular Therapy. 2015;**23**(3):570-577. DOI: 10.1038/mt.2014.226

[71] Maurya AK, Vinayak M. Anticarcinogenic action of quercetin by downregulation of phosphatidylinositol 3-kinase (PI3K) and protein kinase C (PKC) via induction of p53 in hepatocellular carcinoma (HepG2) cell line. Molecular Biology Reports. 2015; **42**(9):1419-1429. DOI: 10.1007/s11033-015-3921-7

[72] Moses C, Nugent F, Waryah CB, et al. Activating PTEN tumor suppressor expression with the CRISPR/dCas9 system. Molecular Therapy - Nucleic Acids. 2019;**14**:287-300. DOI: 10.1016/j.omtn.2018.12.003

[73] Firth AL, Menon T, Parker GS, et al. Functional gene correction for cystic fibrosis in lung epithelial cells generated from patient iPSCs. Cell Reports. 2015; **12**(9):1385-1390. DOI: 10.1016/j.celrep.2015.07.062

[74] Marangi M, Pistritto G. Innovative therapeutic strategies for cystic fibrosis: Moving forward to CRISPR technique. Frontiers in Pharmacology. 2018;**9**:396. DOI: 10.3389/fphar.2018.00396

[75] Shin JW, Kim KH, Chao MJ, et al. Permanent inactivation of Huntington's disease mutation by personalized allele-specific CRISPR/Cas9. Human Molecular Genetics. 2016;**25**(20):4566-4576. DOI: 10.1093/hmg/ddw286

[76] Monteys AM, Ebanks SA, Keiser MS, et al. CRISPR/Cas9 editing of the mutant huntingtin allele *in vitro* and *in vivo*. Molecular Therapy. 2017;**25**(1):12-23. DOI: 10.1016/j.ymthe.2016.11.010

[77] Scharenberg SG, Poletto E, Lucot KL, et al. Engineering monocyte/macrophage-specific glucocerebrosidase expression in human hematopoietic stem cells using genome editing. Nature Communications. 2020;**11**(1):3327. DOI: 10.1038/s41467-020-17148-x

[78] Maxwell KG, Augsornworawat P, Velazco-Cruz L, et al. Gene-edited human stem cell-derived β cells from a patient with monogenic diabetes reverse preexisting diabetes in mice. Science Translational Medicine. 2020;**12**(540): eaax9106. DOI: 10.1126/scitranslmed.aax9106

[79] Christie KA, Robertson LJ, Conway C, et al. Mutation-independent allele-specific editing by CRISPR-Cas9, a novel approach to treat autosomal dominant disease. Molecular Therapy. 2020;**28**(8):1846-1857. DOI: 10.1016/j.ymthe.2020.05.002

[80] Frangoul H, Altshuler D, Cappellini MD, et al. CRISPR-Cas9 gene editing for sickle cell disease and β-thalassemia. The New England Journal of Medicine. 2021;**384**(3):252-260. DOI: 10.1056/NEJMoa2031054

[81] Cwerman-Thibault H, Augustin S, Lechauve C, et al. Nuclear expression of mitochondrial ND4 leads to the protein assembling in complex I and prevents optic atrophy and visual loss. Molecular Therapy - Methods & Clinical Development. 2015;**2**:15003. DOI: 10.1038/mtm.2015.3

[82] Courtney DG, Moore JE, Atkinson SD, et al. CRISPR/Cas9 DNA cleavage at SNP-derived PAM enables both *in vitro* and *in vivo* KRT12 mutation-specific targeting. Gene Therapy. 2016;**23**(1):108-112. DOI: 10.1038/gt.2015.82

[83] Li P, Kleinstiver BP, Leon MY, et al. Allele-specific CRISPR-Cas9 genome editing of the Single-Base P23H mutation for rhodopsin-associated dominant retinitis Pigmentosa. CRISPR Journal. 2018;**1**(1):55-64. DOI: 10.1089/crispr.2017.0009

[84] Amoasii L, Hildyard JCW, Li H, et al. Gene editing restores dystrophin expression in a canine model of Duchenne muscular dystrophy. Science. 2018;**362**(6410):86-91. DOI: 10.1126/science.aau1549

[85] Ekman FK, Ojala DS, Adil MM, et al. CRISPR-Cas9-mediated genome editing increases lifespan and improves motor deficits in a Huntington's disease mouse model. Molecular Therapy - Nucleic Acids. 2019;**17**:829-839. DOI: 10.1016/j.omtn.2019.07.009

[86] Gillmore JD, Gane E, Taubel J, et al. CRISPR-Cas9 *in vivo* gene editing for transthyretin amyloidosis. The New England Journal of Medicine. 2021;**385**(6):493-502. DOI: 10.1056/NEJMoa2107454

[87] Gaj T, Gersbach CA, Barbas CF 3rd. ZFN, TALEN, and CRISPR/Cas-based methods for genome engineering. Trends in Biotechnology. 2013;**31**(7):

397-405. DOI: 10.1016/j.tibtech.2013.04.004

[88] Yanik M, Ponnam SPG, Wimmer T, et al. Development of a reporter system to explore MMEJ in the context of replacing large genomic fragments. Molecular Therapy - Nucleic Acids. 2018;**11**:407-415. DOI: 10.1016/j.omtn.2018.03.010

[89] Kousholt AN, Menzel T, Sørensen CS. Pathways for genome integrity in G2 phase of the cell cycle. Biomolecules. 2012;**2**(4):579-607. DOI: 10.3390/biom2040579

[90] Taleei R, Nikjoo H. Biochemical DSB-repair model for mammalian cells in G1 and early S phases of the cell cycle. Mutation Research. 2013;**756**(1–2): 206-212. DOI: 10.1016/j.mrgentox.2013.06.004

[91] Maruyama T, Dougan SK, Truttmann MC, et al. Increasing the efficiency of precise genome editing with CRISPR-Cas9 by inhibition of nonhomologous end joining. Nature Biotechnology. 2015;**33**(5):538-542. [published correction appears in Nat Biotechnol. 2016 Feb;34(2):210. doi: 10.1038/nbt0216-210c]. DOI: 10.1038/nbt.3190

[92] Li G, Liu D, Zhang X, et al. Suppressing Ku70/Ku80 expression elevates homology-directed repair efficiency in primary fibroblasts. The International Journal of Biochemistry & Cell Biology. 2018;**99**:154-160. DOI: 10.1016/j.biocel.2018.04.011

[93] Wang C, Sun Z, Wang M, et al. Novel CRISPR/Cas9-mediated knockout of LIG4 increases efficiency of site-specific integration in Chinese hamster ovary cell line. Biotechnology Letters. 2022;**44**(9):1063-1072

Chapter 2

Promising New Options for Treating Microbial Keratitis

Faisal Aljassar and Maryam Alsamhan

Abstract

Microbial keratitis is a leading cause of blindness worldwide, estimated up to 5% of the population. There is an increasing incidence of antibiotic resistance, which drives research to find new modalities to treat the disease by targeting the organism's DNA. Using ultraviolet light at different wavelengths at a fixed intensity and duration leads to killing ranges of microorganisms, including bacteria, fungi, and Acanthamoeba. It may be early to compare it to standard treatment; however, it has been shown to be highly effective in managing virulent organisms in animal models. Studies that assess safety and efficacy may also add to the options available to treat microbial keratitis, especially in refractory cases with unknown etiology when there is not much to offer.

Keywords: keratitis, acanthamoeba, ultraviolet corneal cross-linking, bacteria, fungi

1. Introduction

Microbial keratitis is a severe corneal infection that can lead to significant ocular morbidity, including vision loss due to corneal ulceration and scarring, it is the fifth leading cause of blindness worldwide [1]. Traditionally managed with intensive antimicrobial therapies, the rising incidence of drug-resistant pathogens and refractory cases has necessitated the exploration of additional treatment modalities. Corneal cross-linking (CXL), developed initially to treat keratoconus by enhancing corneal biomechanical stability, has emerged as a promising adjunctive therapy for microbial keratitis [2]. The CXL process involves using riboflavin and ultraviolet-A (UV-A) light to induce photochemical reactions that generate reactive oxygen species (ROS) [2]. These ROS not only strengthen the corneal stroma but also exert antimicrobial effects by disrupting microbial cell membranes, DNA, and proteins. Recent research highlights CXL as a viable option, particularly in bacterial infections, where it aids in reducing microbial load and accelerating healing. While it shows variable efficacy in fungal and protozoal infections, ongoing advancements aim to refine CXL protocols by customizing riboflavin formulations, application methods, and combinations with other therapies. As studies continue to assess its safety, efficacy, and integration into clinical practice, CXL holds the potential to significantly enhance the management of resistant and progressive microbial keratitis cases.

2. Corneal cross-linking: A promising approach

Corneal cross-linking is an innovative therapeutic approach that has emerged as a promising option for the management of microbial keratitis [2]. This technique involves the use of ultraviolet light and a photosensitizing agent, typically riboflavin (vitamin B2), to strengthen the corneal stroma and enhance its resistance to infectious agents [2]. By inducing the formation of new covalent bonds between collagen fibrils, CXL has been shown to effectively halt the progression of corneal ectasia and stabilize the corneal structure, thereby improving the eye's natural defense mechanisms against microbial invasion [2]. The application of CXL has demonstrated positive outcomes in the treatment of various forms of microbial keratitis, including those caused by bacteria, fungi, and Acanthamoeba, making it a versatile and valuable tool in the clinician's arsenal against this challenging condition.

Corneal collagen cross-linking (CXL) has demonstrated potential as a treatment for bacterial keratitis in preclinical studies, as shown by a significant reduction in the density and severity of infection in a rat model [3]. The effectiveness of CXL is attributed to its ability to enhance the biomechanical strength of the cornea, making it more resistant to enzymatic degradation by microbial cells [4]. Furthermore, CXL has been observed to potentiate the effects of topical antibiotics, potentially by increasing their penetration into the corneal tissue. However, the efficacy of CXL against fungal infections and its application in herpes simplex keratitis require further investigation [3].

3. Mechanism of action in microbial keratitis

The increasing body of evidence indicates that CXL's dual mechanism—enhancing corneal strength and exerting antimicrobial effects—could be crucial in optimizing treatment strategies for microbial keratitis, particularly in cases where conventional therapies fail or antimicrobial use is restricted due to resistance or adverse effects [4]. Further details on these mechanisms and their clinical implications are provided in **Table 1** below.

Mechanism of action	Description	Benefits
Antimicrobial Effects	• Generation of Reactive Oxygen Species (ROS): CXL generates singlet oxygen and superoxide radicals that damage microbial cells. • Disruption of Cellular Integrity: ROS can directly disrupt the structural components of bacteria, fungi, and some viruses. • Interference with Quorum Sensing: CXL disrupts mechanisms regulating biofilm formation, making microbes more susceptible to antimicrobials. • Enhanced Antibiotic Penetration: CXL can improve antibiotic diffusion into corneal tissues, increasing treatment efficacy.	• Reduces microbial load effectively. • Enhances outcomes of combination therapies against microbial keratitis. • Provides a new approach to managing sight-threatening conditions.

Mechanism of action	Description	Benefits
Biomechanical Stabilization	• Covalent Bond Formation: CXL creates covalent bonds within the corneal stroma. • Strengthening Corneal Structure: Enhances resistance to degradation by infectious agents. • Maintenance of Corneal Integrity: Prevents further damage and complications from microbial keratitis.	• Reduces risk of complications associated with corneal infections. • improved overall corneal stability. • Better visual prognosis for patients with microbial keratitis.

Table 1.
Mechanisms of action of corneal cross-linking (CXL) in microbial keratitis.

4. Indications and considerations for corneal cross-linking (CXL) in microbial keratitis

Corneal cross-linking (CXL) offers a promising alternative or adjunctive treatment approach in several challenging clinical scenarios of microbial keratitis characterized by resistance to standard care or complicated by severe structural issues within the cornea.

4.1 Indications and contraindications for CXL

4.1.1 Indications

4.1.1.1 Resistant infections

CXL is particularly advantageous in cases of microbial keratitis where conventional antibiotic therapies have failed to resolve the infection. This phenomenon is increasingly prevalent with the rise of antimicrobial resistance, which complicates the effective treatment of bacterial, fungal, and some viral infections. The photochemical reactions of CXL generate reactive oxygen species (ROS) that can damage critical cellular components of microbes, potentially overcoming traditional resistance mechanisms [5]. This makes CXL a valuable tool in managing infections that do not respond to antibiotics alone [6].

4.1.1.2 Progressive keratitis

In instances of progressive keratitis—where corneal infection and associated inflammation continue to advance despite ongoing antibiotic therapy—corneal cross-linking can provide significant clinical benefits. The procedure enhances the biomechanical stability of the cornea by promoting covalent bonds within the stroma. This biomechanical reinforcement helps to halt further degradation and thinning of the corneal tissue, which is essential in controlling the progression of severe keratitis [7].

4.1.1.3 Corneal thinning

Significant corneal thinning is a frequent and serious complication of microbial keratitis, increasing the risk of corneal perforation and potential vision loss.

CXL addresses this by reinforcing the structural integrity of the cornea, thus mitigating the risk of further thinning and providing an effective barrier against perforation. By enhancing corneal stability, CXL helps preserve vision and maintain corneal architecture during active infection [8].

While CXL can be a valuable treatment for microbial keratitis, specific contraindications and relative contraindications should be considered:

Contraindications:

- History or suspicion of herpes simplex keratitis: Latent herpes can be reactivated by UV radiation [9].
- Severe keratitis with deeper infiltrates: The standard CXL protocol produces an effective treatment depth limited to 250–300 μm.
- Allergy or hypersensitivity to riboflavin: Any other material used during the procedure may also be a concern.

Relative Contraindications:

- Very thin residual stroma.
- Delayed healing.
- Nystagmus or difficulty with fixating on UV light.
- Pregnancy or nursing.

5. Protocols and variations of CXL

Several protocols and variations of corneal cross-linking (CXL) have been developed to address specific clinical needs in the treatment of microbial keratitis, and these protocols are continuously evolving to enhance efficacy and safety.

5.1 Dresden protocol

The conventional protocol, known as the Dresden Protocol, involves the removal of the corneal epithelium, followed by saturation of the corneal stroma with a riboflavin (vitamin B2) solution. This is achieved by applying a 0.1% isotonic riboflavin solution in 20% dextran every few minutes over a set duration [10]. The cornea is then exposed to ultraviolet-A (UV-A) light at a wavelength of 365 nm with an irradiance of 3 mW/cm^2 for 30 minutes, resulting in a cumulative dose of 5.4 J/cm^2 [10]. This process initiates a photochemical reaction that increases corneal rigidity by forming cross-links within the collagen fibers of the corneal stroma. While effective, this protocol is time-consuming and has led to the development of accelerated protocols that aim to reduce treatment time while maintaining similar outcomes [11].

5.2 Accelerated CXL protocols

Accelerated CXL protocols, such as those used in PACK-CXL (photoactivated chromophores for infectious keratitis), apply higher UV-A irradiances for shorter durations compared to the standard protocol to achieve a similar cumulative energy dose [12]. Accelerated CXL can reduce the overall treatment duration, potentially improving patient convenience and access to the therapy [11, 12].

For example, protocols may use an irradiance of 9 mW/cm^2 for 10 minutes or higher, up to 30 mW/cm^2 for 4 minutes, resulting in a fluence of 7.2 J/cm^2 [11]. While higher irradiances theoretically produce the same photochemical effects by reducing the exposure time, clinical studies have indicated that the biomechanical strengthening effect may diminish at higher intensities [12]. This is possibly due to limitations in oxygen diffusion within the corneal stroma, which is necessary to sustain the chemical reactions that reinforce the corneal structure [13, 14].

Currently, the most common accelerated protocol uses an intensity of 30 mW/cm^2 in continuous light mode for 4 minutes, which equates to a high fluence of 7.2 J/cm^2 [12]. This fluence is applied uniformly across the entire cornea using hypo-osmolar riboflavin, providing a balance between treatment time and efficacy [14].

In addition to varying the intensity and duration of UV-A exposure, different riboflavin formulations have been explored to optimize treatment. Alternatives like hypo-osmolar riboflavin solutions are used to increase corneal penetration in cases where corneal thickness is insufficient. For infectious keratitis, the PACK-CXL protocol specifically utilizes hypo-osmolar riboflavin and varying fluences (e.g., 5.4–7.2 J/cm^2) to effectively treat bacterial and fungal infections, demonstrating comparable success rates to standard antimicrobial therapies [14].

Overall, accelerated protocols and variations in riboflavin formulations offer flexibility in treating microbial keratitis. Current approaches focus on balancing treatment duration, energy dose, and corneal penetration to maximize therapeutic benefits while minimizing side effects and procedural time [13, 14].

5.3 PACK-CXL

PACK-CXL (Photoactivated Chromophore for Keratitis-Cross-Linking) follows the Bunsen-Roscoe law of reciprocity, which implies that the effectiveness of light in inducing photochemical reactions depends on the total energy exposure, considering both intensity and time [15]. Many studies have shown varied outcomes regarding the efficacy of PACK-CXL [16–27]. Recent studies suggest that accelerated PACK-CXL could be clinically efficient compared to the standard Dresden protocol when careful modifications are made regarding the type of pathogen present in the cornea in order to maintain an appropriate killing rate [28]. Although PACK-CXL has proven ineffective for treating viral or Acanthamoeba keratitis and has even been reported to reactivate herpes simplex virus infections potentially, it has been suggested that it may be beneficial for bacterial and fungal keratitis, either as a stand-alone treatment or as a supplement to antimicrobial medications [2, 28]. Recent studies have confirmed that PACK-CXL has beneficial antimicrobial efficacy, especially for moderate ulcers [28].

PACK-CXL now requires further protocol modifications to tailor treatment to specific pathogens or clinical situations. Adjustments in treatment parameters—such as irradiation duration, type of chromophore, and fluence used—might help enhance the microbicidal efficiency of PACK-CXL based on the specific type of pathogen being targeted [29].

These protocol variations and advancements in CXL technology have enabled clinicians to tailor the treatment to the specific needs of patients with microbial keratitis, offering more personalized and efficient management strategies.

Type of keratitis	Efficacy of CXL	Key points
Bacterial Keratitis	CXL shows significant promise against common pathogens, particularly Staphylococcus aureus and Pseudomonas aeruginosa.	• Improved infection resolution rates. • Reduced healing times. • Fewer complications compared to standard antimicrobial therapy alone [13].
Fungal Keratitis	Efficacy in fungal infections is variable; some studies report reduced fungal load while others find minimal impact, especially against filamentous fungi like Fusarium.	• Thick fungal cell walls may protect against UV-A light, limiting CXL's effectiveness [14]. • PACK-CXL offers a cost-effective alternative to traditional antifungal agents. • Potentially facilitates faster recovery for noncompliant patients due to lower treatment costs.
Acanthamoeba Keratitis	CXL has limited efficacy against Acanthamoeba, especially in its cystic form, which is resistant to UV-A light and ROS.	• Generally, it is not recommended as a stand-alone therapy. • Can provide some biomechanical stabilization to the cornea [14].
Viral Keratitis	CXL's role in viral keratitis, such as that caused by herpes simplex virus (HSV), is still under investigation.	• May not directly target the viral pathogen. • Suggested to improve corneal integrity and reduce scarring in chronic herpes keratitis cases. • Some studies indicate potential benefits in healing rates and reducing episodes of viral recurrence, requiring further research for definitive efficacy [13].

Table 2.
Efficacy of corneal cross-linking (CXL) in treating different types of microbial keratitis.

6. Efficacy of CXL in different types of microbial keratitis

Corneal cross-linking (CXL) has emerged as a promising treatment, particularly in cases resistant to traditional therapies. The efficacy of CXL can vary depending on the specific type of microbial keratitis being treated. Further information on the effectiveness of CXL across different types of microbial keratitis is provided in **Table 2**.

Overall, the role of CXL in microbial keratitis is still under rigorous investigation. Still, preliminary results indicate that it can be a valuable adjunctive therapy that augments the effectiveness of conventional treatments across various microbial infections.

7. Clinical outcomes and safety

Corneal cross-linking (CXL) has gained traction as a viable therapeutic option for strengthening the corneal stroma in conditions such as keratoconus and post-LASIK ectasia [30]. The procedure involves the application of riboflavin (vitamin B2) followed by ultraviolet-A (UV-A) irradiation, which leads to the formation of covalent bonds between collagen fibers in the cornea, thereby increasing its stiffness and potentially halting the progression of corneal ectasia [30].

Studies have consistently reported favorable clinical outcomes following CXL treatment, demonstrating significant reductions in corneal curvature and improvements in uncorrected visual acuity (UCVA) post-procedure. The healing outcomes after CXL vary depending on the context in which it is performed, but many patients achieve stable and improved visual outcomes over time [30]. Research shows that a majority of patients experience an improvement in best-corrected visual acuity (BCVA), with many retaining or achieving functional vision [31]. The clinical outcomes of CXL in the treatment of microbial keratitis have also been encouraging, with several studies reporting significant improvements in visual acuity, reductions in corneal scarring, and prevention of vision-threatening complications such as corneal perforation [30]. Moreover, current studies suggest that CXL may reduce corneal neovascularization and lymphatics, which could increase the success rate of high-risk keratoplasty grafts.

A recent prospective randomized trial comparing photoactivated chromophore corneal cross-linking (PACK-CXL) to standard antimicrobial therapy for bacterial, fungal, and mixed infectious keratitis found that both treatments led to similar visual acuity outcomes over time. At the final follow-up, there were no significant differences between the two groups in terms of both uncorrected and corrected distance visual acuity, suggesting that PACK-CXL is as effective as standard antimicrobial therapy in preserving and improving visual acuity in patients with infectious keratitis [14].

CXL has been shown to be a safe procedure when performed by experienced clinicians. The most common adverse effects include mild eye discomfort, sensitivity to light, and temporary corneal haze, which usually resolves within a few weeks after treatment [4]. Serious complications, such as corneal infection, damage to the corneal endothelium, or significant visual impairment, are rare when the procedure is performed according to established protocols and guidelines [4].

Overall, the clinical evidence supports the use of CXL as a safe and effective treatment option for managing various types of microbial keratitis, particularly in cases where conventional therapies have been ineffective or when the cornea is at risk of further deterioration. Proper patient selection, adherence to treatment protocols, and close monitoring are crucial to ensure optimal outcomes and minimize the risk of complications.

8. Studies and meta-analyses

In vitro and ex vivo studies play a crucial role in advancing the understanding of corneal cross-linking (CXL) and its mechanisms of action. These studies provide valuable insights into how CXL can effectively strengthen the corneal structure and enhance its resistance to biochemical and mechanical stress.

8.1 In vitro studies

In vitro studies have explored the effects of corneal cross-linking (CXL) on corneal tissues to assess biochemical and biomechanical changes. For example, studies by Wollensak et al. and Spoerl et al. exposed keratocytes to riboflavin and UV-A light, demonstrating that the CXL process significantly increases the stiffness of the corneal tissue while also inducing a cytotoxic effect on keratocytes, particularly at higher UV-A doses, which is a crucial consideration for the safety of the CXL procedure. Furthermore, research indicates that CXL treatment enhances the resistance of corneal stromal cells to enzymatic digestion by proteolytic enzymes, thereby suggesting an increase in corneal stability and durability after the procedure [32].

8.2 Ex vivo studies

Ex vivo studies have been employed to evaluate the safety and effects of corneal cross-linking (CXL) on corneal epithelial cells in conditions that closely mimic the physiological environment. For example, a study by Shetty et al. investigated the effects of accelerated corneal cross-linking (ACXL) compared to conventional CXL on ex vivo-cultured limbal epithelial cells. The findings demonstrated that ACXL, which uses a higher UV-A irradiance for a shorter duration, results in less cellular apoptosis compared to the standard CXL protocol, highlighting its potential safety advantages in clinical settings. The study showed that higher intensity UV-A exposure for a shorter period (30 mW/cm^2 for 3 minutes) was associated with significantly lower cell death compared to lower intensity exposure for a more extended period (3 mW/cm^2 for 30 minutes), suggesting that ACXL may provide a safer alternative with reduced cellular damage [33].

Additionally, the research highlighted that the use of riboflavin during CXL mitigates the adverse effects on limbal epithelial cells, enhancing cell survival and potentially supporting better corneal healing outcomes. The study also emphasizes the importance of understanding the molecular and cellular responses to different CXL protocols to establish safe treatment parameters [33].

8.3 Comparative studies

Comparative studies often focus on evaluating different CXL protocols, such as standard (C-CXL) versus accelerated (A-CXL) cross-linking, to determine their relative efficacy. A meta-analysis by Shajari et al. compared the clinical outcomes of C-CXL and A-CXL in patients with progressive keratoconus, demonstrating that both methods are effective in strengthening corneal tissue. However, C-CXL was superior in terms of achieving more significant reductions in minimum keratometric values and a deeper demarcation line, suggesting higher treatment efficacy, while A-CXL was associated with less corneal thinning, indicating potential safety benefits [34].

8.4 Meta-analyses

Meta-analyses that combine data from multiple studies provide robust evidence for the safety and effectiveness of CXL. A systematic review and meta-analysis by Tian et al. examined the impact of CXL on patients with keratoconus, finding consistent improvements in uncorrected and best-corrected visual acuity (UCVA and BCVA) and stabilization of corneal topography over long-term follow-up. This study underscored the low complication rate associated with CXL, reinforcing its role as a primary treatment for keratoconus and other corneal ectasias [35].

Furthermore, another meta-analysis highlighted that while both C-CXL and A-CXL provide effective outcomes, the choice between these protocols may depend on individual patient factors and the desired balance between efficacy and safety. For instance, A-CXL, which involves shorter irradiation times, may reduce the risk of intraoperative complications and be more convenient for patients and clinicians [34].

Overall, comparative studies and meta-analyses offer valuable insights into the clinical effectiveness of CXL, informing best practices, guiding patient selection, and shaping the ongoing evolution of treatment protocols for corneal disorders. Such research is essential for optimizing patient care and improving outcomes associated with CXL treatment.

9. Future directions

The future of corneal cross-linking (CXL) holds exciting possibilities that can enhance its applications and effectiveness in treating corneal disorders. One significant trend in the evolution of CXL is the development of accelerated techniques that utilize shorter UV-A exposure times with increased irradiance [12]. Ongoing research aims to refine these accelerated methods, which have shown promise in delivering comparable or even superior outcomes in terms of corneal rigidity and visual acuity. By minimizing treatment time, these methods may enhance patient comfort and make CXL more accessible to a broader range of individuals [12].

9.1 Combining CXL with other treatments

Another critical direction for CXL includes exploring its integration with other therapeutic modalities. Combining CXL with advanced surgical techniques, such as femtosecond laser-assisted procedures, could further stabilize the cornea and improve visual outcomes [36]. Additionally, research is underway to examine the benefits of pairing CXL with pharmacological treatments, to address corneal neovascularization—a significant challenge in achieving successful grafts in high-risk keratoplasty patients [37, 38]. These combination therapies may lead to improved healing and enhanced overall effectiveness of corneal treatments.

9.2 Protocol optimization

Optimizing the protocols used in CXL procedures is vital for maximizing treatment outcomes. This includes determining the ideal riboflavin formulation, application techniques, and UV exposure parameters [39, 40]. Standardizing these protocols can potentially reduce variability in treatment outcomes and promote more predictable results across different patient populations. As new formulations and technologies emerge, ongoing research will focus on refining these protocols to improve safety and efficacy.

9.3 Personalized approaches

As our understanding of the biology of the cornea and individual patient variations improves, there is potential for personalized CXL approaches. By considering factors such as the specific corneal condition, patient age, and overall eye health, tailored CXL treatments could optimize results and minimize complications [39, 40]. This approach may include customizing treatment protocols and follow-up care based on individual responses to therapy, thereby enhancing the effectiveness of CXL for diverse patient populations.

Moreover, while CXL is well-established for conditions like keratoconus and post-LASIK ectasia, expanding its indications to include other corneal diseases, such as infectious keratitis and corneal dystrophies, represents a crucial area of exploration [40]. Ongoing clinical trials aim to assess the safety and efficacy of CXL in these new patient populations, focusing on identifying appropriate candidates and tailoring treatment protocols for diverse corneal conditions.

Innovations in biomaterials and drug delivery systems are also set to revolutionize CXL procedures. The development of new riboflavin formulations that enhance corneal absorption, combined with biodegradable polymers that allow for sustained release of therapeutic agents post-CXL, may significantly improve treatment outcomes [41]. These advancements could lead to more effective procedures, reduced side effects, and faster recovery times for patients.

The development of robust clinical guidelines and standardized protocols for CXL is essential, especially as new techniques and indications emerge. Establishing evidence-based guidelines will ensure consistency in practice and promote optimal patient outcomes across diverse clinical settings. Ongoing collaboration among researchers, practitioners, and regulatory bodies will be crucial to developing these frameworks and contributing to best practices in the field.

Finally, future research will concentrate on longitudinal studies to assess the long-term safety and effectiveness of CXL in various patient populations. This type of research will provide essential data to inform best practices and help clinicians make evidence-based decisions about patient management.

In conclusion, the future directions of corneal cross-linking are filled with potential advancements that can enhance its role in corneal health management. By exploring new techniques, expanding treatment indications, utilizing innovative materials, optimizing protocols, and developing personalized approaches, CXL has the opportunity to improve patient outcomes for a variety of corneal disorders significantly. These advancements not only promise to elevate the standard of care but also to redefine the landscape of corneal treatments for patients and practitioners alike.

10. Conclusion

10.1 Advancing the management of microbial keratitis

Corneal cross-linking (CXL) represents a significant advancement in the treatment of microbial keratitis, offering a multifaceted approach that combines biomechanical stabilization with antimicrobial efficacy. The insights gained from understanding the mechanisms of action, including the generation of reactive oxygen species and the enhancement of traditional antimicrobial therapies, have positioned CXL as a vital tool in the ophthalmologist's repertoire. As microbial resistance continues to rise, the role of CXL in managing resistant and progressive forms of keratitis is increasingly critical.

The exploration of various protocols, including the standard Dresden Protocol and newer methods like accelerated CXL, transepithelial CXL, and PACK-CXL, demonstrates the versatility of this treatment. Each approach can be tailored to meet the specific needs of patients, thus enhancing treatment outcomes and promoting better patient compliance. Additionally, the incorporation of advanced techniques and personalized strategies into future research has the potential to optimize CXL's application further, ensuring its relevance in an evolving therapeutic landscape.

As ongoing studies evaluate the long-term safety and effectiveness of CXL, there is hope for establishing standard guidelines that maximize its benefits while minimizing risks. The future of microbial keratitis management lies in the continued innovation and refinement of CXL protocols aimed at creating a comprehensive, evidence-based framework that enhances patient outcomes and addresses the complexities of various corneal diseases. Overall, the advancements in CXL not only promise improved standards of care for patients but also signify a transformative shift in the management of microbial infections affecting the cornea.

Acknowledgements

This manuscript was written with the aid of Artificial intelligence, namely ChatGPT, in grammar checking and paraphrasing, working in accordance with IntechOpen authorship policy.

The content has been reviewed and verified by the authors to ensure accuracy and compliance with ethical writing standards. Further, the authors declare that there is no conflict of interest and no funding was received.

Nomenclature

CXL	corneal cross-linking
PACK-CXL	photoactivated chromophore for infectious keratitis corneal cross-linking
UV-A	ultraviolet-A
J/cm^2	joules per square centimeter
mW/cm^2	milliwatts per square centimeter
ROS	reactive oxygen species
HPMC	hydroxypropyl methylcellulose
UCVA	uncorrected visual acuity
BCVA	best-corrected visual acuity

Author details

Faisal Aljassar[1*] and Maryam Alsamhan[2]

1 Ministry of Health, Alsalam International Hospital and Kuwait Oil Company Hospital, Kuwait City, Kuwait

2 Ministry of Health, Kuwait City, Kuwait

*Address all correspondence to: faialjassar@gmail.com

References

[1] Cabrera-Aguas M, Khoo P, Watson SL. Infectious keratitis: A review. Clinical and Experimental Ophthalmology. 2022;**50**(5):543-562. DOI: 10.1111/ceo.14113

[2] Price MO, Tenkman LR, Schrier A, Fairchild KM, Trokel SL, Price FW. Photoactivated riboflavin treatment of infectious keratitis using collagen cross-linking technology. Journal of Refractive Surgery. 2012;**28**(10):706-713. DOI: 10.3928/1081597X-20120921-06

[3] Kilic BB, Altiörs D, Demirbilek M, Ogus E. Comparison between corneal cross-linking, topical antibiotic and combined therapy in experimental bacterial keratitis model. Saudi Journal of Ophthalmology. 2018;**32**:97-104. DOI: 10.1016/j.sjopt.2017.10.003

[4] Naranjo A, Manche EE. A comprehensive review on corneal crosslinking. Taiwan Journal of Ophthalmology. 2024;**14**(1):44-49. DOI: 10.4103/tjo.TJO-D-23-00055

[5] Alio JL, Abbouda A, Diaz Valle D, Benitez del Castillo JM, Gegundez Fernandez JA. Corneal cross linking and infectious keratitis: A systematic review with a meta-analysis of reported cases. Journal of Ophthalmic Inflammation and Infection. 2013;**3**:47. DOI: 10.1186/1869-5760-3-47

[6] Richoz O, Hammer A, Tabibian D, Gatzioufas Z, Hafezi F. The biomechanical effect of corneal collagen cross-linking (CXL) with riboflavin and UV-A is oxygen dependent. Translational Vision Science and Technology. 2013;**2**(7):6. DOI: 10.1167/tvst.2.7.6

[7] Mazzotta C, Caporossi T, Denaro R, Bovone C, Sparano C, Paradiso A, et al. Morphological and functional correlations in riboflavin UV a corneal collagen cross-linking for keratoconus. Acta Ophthalmologica. 2012;**90**:259-265. DOI: 10.1111/j.1755-3768.2010.01890.x

[8] Meek KM, Hayes S. Corneal cross-linking – A review. Ophthalmic and Physiological Optics. 2013;**33**:78-93. DOI: 10.1111/opo.12032

[9] Sitaula S, Singh SK, Gurung A. Bilateral viral keratitis following corneal collagen crosslinking for progressive keratoconus. Journal of Ophthalmic Inflammation and Infection. 2019;**9**:16. DOI: 10.1186/s12348-019-0185-8

[10] Vandevenne MMS, Berendschot TTJM, Visser N, Dickman MM, Nuijts RMMA. Late-onset corneal edema after customized crosslinking for progressive keratoconus. American Journal of Ophthalmology Case Reports. 2024;**102090**:2-5. DOI: 10.1016/j.ajoc.2024.102090

[11] Hafezi NL, Aydemir ME, Lu NJ, Torres-Netto EA, Hillen M, Koppen C. Effect of accelerated high-fluence riboflavin and rose bengal-mediated corneal cross-linking on resistance to enzymatic digestion. BMC Ophthalmology. 2024;**24**:32. DOI: 10.1186/s12886-024-03293-0

[12] Kandel H, Abbondanza M, Gupta A, et al. Comparison of standard versus accelerated corneal collagen cross-linking for keratoconus: 5-year outcomes from the save sight keratoconus registry. Eye. 2024;**38**:95-102. DOI: 10.1038/s41433-023-02641-6

[13] Mazzotta C, Baiocchi S, Denaro R, et al. Optical coherence tomography and confocal microscopy following three different protocols of corneal

collagen-crosslinking in keratoconus. Investigative Ophthalmology and Visual Science. 2014;**55**(11):7601-7609. DOI: 10.1167/iovs.14-14888

[14] Hafezi F, Hosny M, Shetty R, Knyazer B, Chen S, Wang Q, et al. PACK-CXL vs. antimicrobial therapy for bacterial, fungal, and mixed infectious keratitis: A prospective randomized phase 3 trial. Eye and Vision (London). 2022;**9**:2. DOI: 10.1186/s40662-021-00272-0

[15] Hafezi F, Randleman JB. PACK-CXL: Defining CXL for infectious keratitis. Journal of Refractive Surgery. 2014;**30**(7):438-439. DOI: 10.3928/1081597X-20140609-01

[16] Panda A, Krishna SN, Kumar S. Photo-activated riboflavin therapy of refractory corneal ulcers. Cornea. 2012;**31**(10):1210-1213. DOI: 10.1097/ICO.0b013e31823f8f48

[17] Müller L, Thiel MA, Kipfer-Kauer AI, Kaufmann C. Corneal cross-linking as supplementary treatment option in melting keratitis: A case series. Klinische Monatsblätter für Augenheilkunde. 2012;**229**(4):411-415. DOI: 10.1055/s-0031-1299420

[18] Li Z, Jhanji V, Tao X, Yu H, Chen W, Mu G. Riboflavin/ultraviolet light-mediated crosslinking for fungal keratitis. The British Journal of Ophthalmology. 2013;**97**(5):669-671. DOI: 10.1136/bjophthalmol-2012-302518

[19] Sorkhabi R, Sedgipoor M, Mahdavifard A. Collagen cross-linking for resistant corneal ulcer. International Ophthalmology. 2013;**33**(1):61-66. DOI: 10.1007/s10792-012-9633-2

[20] Tabibian D, Richoz O, Riat A, Schrenzel J, Hafezi F. Accelerated photoactivated chromophore for keratitis-corneal collagen cross-linking as a first-line and sole treatment in early fungal keratitis. Journal of Refractive Surgery. 2014;**30**(12):855-857. DOI: 10.3928/1081597X-20141113-06

[21] Said DG, Elalfy MS, Gatzioufas Z, et al. Collagen cross-linking with photoactivated riboflavin (PACK-CXL) for the treatment of advanced infectious keratitis with corneal melting. Ophthalmology. 2014;**121**(7):1377-1382. DOI: 10.1016/j.ophtha.2014.01.011

[22] Shetty R, Nagaraja H, Jayadev C, Shivanna Y, Kugar T. Collagen crosslinking in the management of advanced non-resolving microbial keratitis. The British Journal of Ophthalmology. 2014;**98**(8):1033-1035. DOI: 10.1136/bjophthalmol-2014-304944

[23] Vajpayee RB, Shafi SN, Maharana PK, Sharma N, Jhanji V. Evaluation of corneal collagen cross-linking as an additional therapy in mycotic keratitis. Clinical and Experimental Ophthalmology. 2015;**43**(2):103-107. DOI: 10.1111/ceo.12399

[24] Uddaraju M, Mascarenhas J, Das MR, et al. Corneal cross-linking as an adjuvant therapy in the management of recalcitrant deep stromal fungal keratitis: A randomized trial. American Journal of Ophthalmology. 2015;**160**(1):131-4.e5. DOI: 10.1016/j.ajo.2015.03.024

[25] Igal V, Pikkel Igal YS, Pikkel YY. Corneal cross-linking as a treatment for fungal keratitis associated with corneal melting. Case Reports in Ophthalmology. 2017;**8**(1):148-151. DOI: 10.1159/000456537

[26] Erdem E, Harbiyeli II, Boral H, Ilkit M, Yagmur M, Ersoz R. Corneal collagen cross-linking for the management of mycotic keratitis.

Mycopathologia. 2018;**183**(3):521-527. DOI: 10.1007/s11046-018-0247-8

[27] Prajna NV, Radhakrishnan N, Lalitha P, et al. Cross-linking-assisted infection reduction: A randomized clinical trial evaluating the effect of adjuvant cross-linking on outcomes in fungal keratitis. Ophthalmology. 2020;**127**(2):159-166. DOI: 10.1016/j.ophtha.2019.08.029

[28] Awad R, Ghaith AA, Awad K, Saad MM, Elmassry AA. Fungal keratitis: Diagnosis, management, and recent advances. Clinical Ophthalmology. 2024;**18**:85-106. DOI: 10.2147/OPTH.S447138

[29] Ting DSJ, Henein C, Said DG, Dua HS. Photoactivated chromophore for infectious keratitis - Corneal cross-linking (PACK-CXL): A systematic review and meta-analysis. The Ocular Surface. 2019;**17**(4):624-634. DOI: doi.org/10.1016/j.jtos.2019.08.006

[30] Amaral DC, Menezes AHG, Vilaça Lima LC, Faneli AC, Neto PFS, Canedo ALC, et al. Corneal collagen crosslinking for ectasia after refractive surgery: A systematic review and meta-analysis. Clinical Ophthalmology. 2024;**18**:865-879. DOI: 10.2147/OPTH.S451232

[31] Kodavoor SK, Sarwate NJ, Ramamurhy D. Microbial keratitis following accelerated corneal collagen cross-linking. Oman Journal of Ophthalmology. 2015;**8**(2):111-113. DOI: 10.4103/0974-620X.159259

[32] Spoerl E, Hoyer A, Pillunat LE, Raiskup F. Corneal cross-linking and safety issues. The Open Ophthalmology Journal. 2011;**5**:14-16

[33] Shetty R, Matalia H, Nuijts R, Subramani M, Dhamodaran K, Pandian R, et al. Safety profile of accelerated corneal cross-linking versus conventional cross-linking: A comparative study on ex vivo-cultured limbal epithelial cells. The British Journal of Ophthalmology. 2015;**99**(2):272-280. DOI: 10.1136/bjophthalmol-2014-305495

[34] Shajari M, Kolb CM, Agha B, Steinwender G, Müller M, Herrmann E, et al. Comparison of standard and accelerated corneal cross-linking for the treatment of keratoconus: A meta-analysis. Acta Ophthalmologica. 2019;**97**:7-13. DOI: 10.1111/aos.13814

[35] Tian C, Xiujun P, Zhengjun F, Xia Z, Feihu Z. Corneal collagen cross-linking in keratoconus: A systematic review and meta-analysis. Scientific Reports. 2014;**4**:5652. DOI: 10.1038/srep05652

[36] Mazzotta C, Zagari M, Bona G, Ponzin D, Awwad ST, Torres-Netto EA, et al. Crosslinked all-femtosecond laser-cut corneal allogenic intracorneal ring segments (AFXL CAIRSs): Pilot ex vivo study and report of first two cases performed in Italy. Journal of Clinical Medicine. 2024;**13**(19):5771. DOI: 10.3390/jcm13195771

[37] Schaub F, Hou Y, Zhang W, Bock F, Hos D, Cursiefen C. Corneal crosslinking to regress pathologic corneal neovascularization before high-risk keratoplasty. Cornea. 2021;**40**(2):147-155. DOI: 10.1097/ICO.0000000000002406

[38] Lu N-J, Hafezi F, Koppen C, Aslanides IM. Editorial: Research and advances on medication for corneal diseases and surgery. Frontiers in Pharmacology. 2024;**15**:1434180. DOI: 10.3389/fphar.2024.1434180

[39] Angelo L, Boptom AG, McGhee C, Ziaei M. Corneal crosslinking: Present and future. The Asia-Pacific Journal of

Ophthalmology. 2022;**11**(5):441-452. DOI: 10.1097/APO.0000000000000557

[40] Deshmukh R, Ong ZZ, Rampat R, Alió del Barrio JL, Barua A, Ang M, et al. Management of keratoconus: An updated review. Frontiers in Medicine. 2023;**10**:1212314. DOI: 10.3389/fmed.2023.1212314

[41] Ting DS. Current and emerging therapies for corneal infection: A clinical and laboratory study [Dissertation]. Nottingham: University of Nottingham; 2022. DOI: 10.13140/RG.2.2.36250.01288

Chapter 3

Retinal Organoids: Advances in Generation, Development, and Applications – From Stem Cells to Disease Modeling and Regenerative Medicine

Reyhaneh Sadat Mousavi, Fatemeh Naghshnejad,
Fereshteh Karamali and Leila Satarian

Abstract

Retinal diseases, often caused by the degeneration of light-sensitive cells, pose a significant global health challenge. While current treatments are limited, cell therapy, involving the transplantation of healthy cells, offers hope. Recent advancements in stem cell technology have enabled the creation of 3D retinal organoids, which closely mimic the structure and function of the human retina. These organoids provide a valuable platform for studying retinal development, modeling diseases, and testing potential therapies. By understanding the molecular mechanisms underlying eye formation and disease progression, researchers can identify and develop targeted treatments. Retinal organoids hold the promise of revolutionizing the field of regenerative medicine and vision research, offering hope for restoring vision and improving the lives of individuals affected by retinal diseases.

Keywords: retinal organoid, pluripotent stem cells, retinal diseases, cell therapy, regenerative medicine

1. Introduction

Vision is one of the most vital senses through which we interact with our environment, allowing us to perceive and interpret the world around us. Any disorder that disrupts the transmission of visual signals to the sensitive retinal layer is classified as a vision disorder. Such impairments not only affect individuals but also have significant economic and social repercussions for society as a whole [1].

In mammals, including humans, the retinal layer possesses limited regenerative capacity. Consequently, severe damage to retinal cells can lead to significant vision impairment and, ultimately, blindness. Despite extensive research into various therapeutic strategies, a definitive treatment for retinal cell degeneration remains elusive.

Over the past three decades, the field of cell therapy has emerged as a promising avenue for addressing retinal damage by supporting/replacing lost or dysfunctional cells with healthy ones. Initial studies utilized primary retinal cells derived from aborted embryos, revealing that photoreceptor progenitor cells—young cells that have exited the cell division cycle are particularly effective in restoring function in damaged retinas [1].

Research has demonstrated that transplanted photoreceptor cells can aid recovery in injured models through two primary mechanisms: by sharing cytoplasmic components with host cells to protect them from further damage, or by directly replacing the lost cells in the host retina [2, 3]. However, ethical concerns surrounding the use of cells derived from aborted embryos have prompted the exploration of alternative sources. The advent of embryonic pluripotent stem cells (ESCs) and induced pluripotent stem cells (iPSCs), which possess remarkable proliferation and differentiation capabilities, has provided a viable alternative for cell therapy research.

A pivotal development in this field has been the establishment of cell culture conditions that facilitate the generation of 3D organoid structures from pluripotent stem cells. These organoids closely mimic the *in vivo* environment, offering a unique platform for studying human retinal development and function. The ability to recreate the conditions of human development in the laboratory not only enhances our understanding of retinal biology but also allows for large-scale drug evaluation and disease modeling.

In recent years, numerous studies have focused on optimizing differentiation methods to generate retinal organoids from various cell types, as well as identifying the factors that enhance their efficiency. This chapter will first explore the stages of natural retinal development, followed by a detailed examination of the methodologies for deriving retinal organoids from different cell sources. Additionally, we will discuss modern technologies that minimize individual variability in cultivation methods, thereby improving the simulation of physiological conditions. Finally, we will highlight the applications of retinal organoids in disease modeling and drug screening, underscoring their potential to transform our approach to understanding and treating retinal disorders.

2. The intricate world of retinal development

2.1 Anatomy and structure of the retina

The eye is one of the most complex and vital sensory organs in living organisms, primarily responsible for receiving, processing, and interpreting light signals, which are then converted into chemical messages transmitted to the visual center of the brain. The eyeball is composed of three distinct layers: the outer layer (sclera), the middle layer (choroid), and the inner layer (retina) (**Figure 1**) [4].

The sclera, rich in collagen, serves as a protective barrier against both external and internal pressures. At the front of the eye, the sclera becomes transparent, forming the cornea, which allows light to enter the eye. The cornea covers the iris, pupil, and aqueous humor, playing a crucial role in light transmission. The choroid, the middle layer of the eye, is essential for supplying blood and nutrients to the ocular structures.

The iris features a central pupil whose diameter adjusts in response to the contraction of iris muscles, thereby regulating the amount of light entering the eye. Additionally, the ciliary body, located at the junction of the choroid and iris, controls the shape of the lens by contracting its associated muscles.

The retina, the innermost layer of the eye, is primarily responsible for converting light signals into neural impulses that are sent to the brain for interpretation. This layer contains over seven distinct cell types, each playing a critical role in the visual process. The outermost cells, closest to the choroid, are known as retinal pigment epithelium (RPE) cells, which are non-neuronal in nature. RPE cells are integral to the formation of the blood-retinal barrier due to their strong intercellular connections [5].

Adjacent to the apical membrane of RPE cells are the cylindrical (rod) and cone photoreceptor cells, with their cell bodies located in the outer nuclear layer (ONL). The outer segments of these photoreceptors form synapses with the dendrites of bipolar and horizontal cells in the outer plexiform layer (OPL). The nuclei of these interneurons reside in the inner nuclear layer (INL) and synapse with ganglion cells in the inner plexiform layer (IPL). The axonal projections of ganglion cells converge to form the optic nerve, transmitting visual information to the brain. Additionally, Müller glial cells extend throughout the retinal layer, providing structural support and maintaining retinal homeostasis (**Figure 1**) [4].

This intricate organization of the retina not only highlights its complexity but also underscores the critical interplay between its various cell types in the process of vision. Understanding these anatomical and structural details is essential for advancing research in retinal development and the application of retinal organoids in therapeutic contexts.

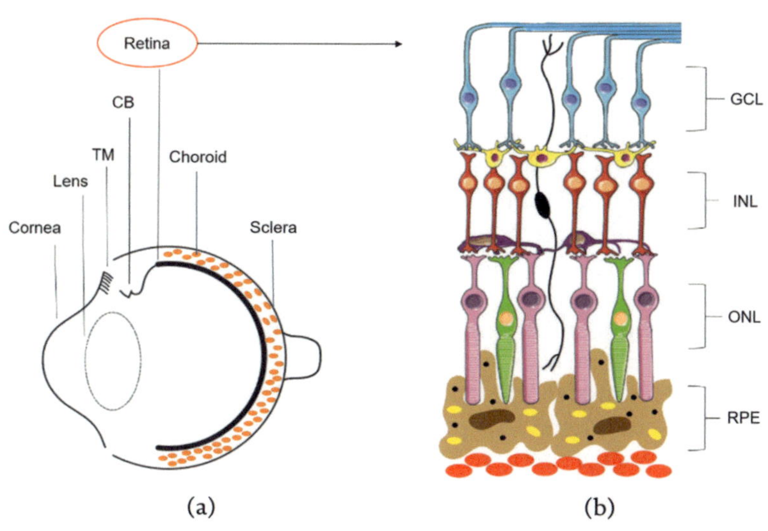

Figure 1.
(A) This schematic illustration demonstrates that the eyeball is made up of three distinct layers: sclera, choroid, and retina. (B) The retina, which is the innermost layer of the eye, comprises more than seven different cell types, each essential for the visual process. The outermost cells, adjacent to the choroid, are referred to as retinal pigment epithelium (RPE) cells. The outer nuclear layer (ONL) contains the nuclei of photoreceptors, while the inner nuclear layer (INL) houses the nuclei of various retinal neural cells, including amacrine, bipolar, and horizontal cells. The retinal ganglion cells layer (GCL) consists of ganglion cells and their axons.

2.2 Retinal development

During embryonic development, the eye region originates from the anterior neural ectoderm. As brain development progresses, the surface ectoderm transforms into neural ectoderm in response to inhibitory signals derived from the notochord and paraxial mesoderm [6]. The neural ectoderm then separates from the surface ectoderm and begins to thicken, first forming a neural plate and subsequently a neural groove that invaginates inward until it differentiates into a neural tube, distinct from the overlying surface ectoderm.

Concurrent with the development of the neural tube, other tissues derived from the mesoderm and endoderm also begin to form. The simultaneous interactions between these structures lead to the commitment of cells toward an anterior neural fat; see **Figure 2**.

The distal region of the vesicles interacts with the overlying lens ectoderm, which subsequently leads to the formation of the lens placode. This interaction induces the invagination of both the lens placode and the distal optic vesicles, resulting in the development of optic cups [3]. At least five essential signaling pathways play a role in eye patterning: (i) fibroblast growth factors (FGF1 and FGF2), (ii) transforming growth factor beta (TGFβ), (iii) bone morphogenetic protein (BMP), (iv) Wnt, and (v) Sonic hedgehog (Shh) [5].

The formation of the eye field is marked by the expression of specific genes, including paired box 6 (PAX6), paired-type homeodomain transcription factor (RAX, previously known as RX), SIX homeobox 3 (SIX3), and SIX6. The development of optic vesicles features the expression of orthodenticle homeobox 2 protein (OTX2), the paired-like homeodomain transcription factor (VSX2, formerly CHX10), and microphthalmia-associated transcription factor (MITF). Generally, cells in the optic vesicle are bipotent, capable of differentiating into both neural retina and RPE. The fate of these cells is determined by a specific time frame for the local expression of MITF and VSX2.

As the development of the retina continues, the neural retina further differentiates into various cell types essential for visual function, such as photoreceptors, bipolar cells, horizontal cells, amacrine cells, and ganglion cells. These cells align to form the distinctive layered structure of the mature retina, with photoreceptors situated in the outer nuclear layer, interneurons in the inner nuclear layer, and ganglion cells in the ganglion cell layer.

A comprehensive understanding of the complex process of retinal development—from the formation of the optic vesicle to the establishment of mature retinal cell types—is vital for modeling retinal development *in vitro* using retinal organoids. By mimicking these developmental processes, retinal organoids can provide valuable insights into the molecular mechanisms of retinal specification and differentiation, as well as offer a platform for studying retinal diseases and exploring potential treatments.

3. Pioneering retinal organoid generation

3.1 Historical perspectives on retinal organoid research

The term "retinal organoid" was first introduced in 2013 to describe cell aggregates derived from pluripotent stem cells [8]. The schematic timeline of key

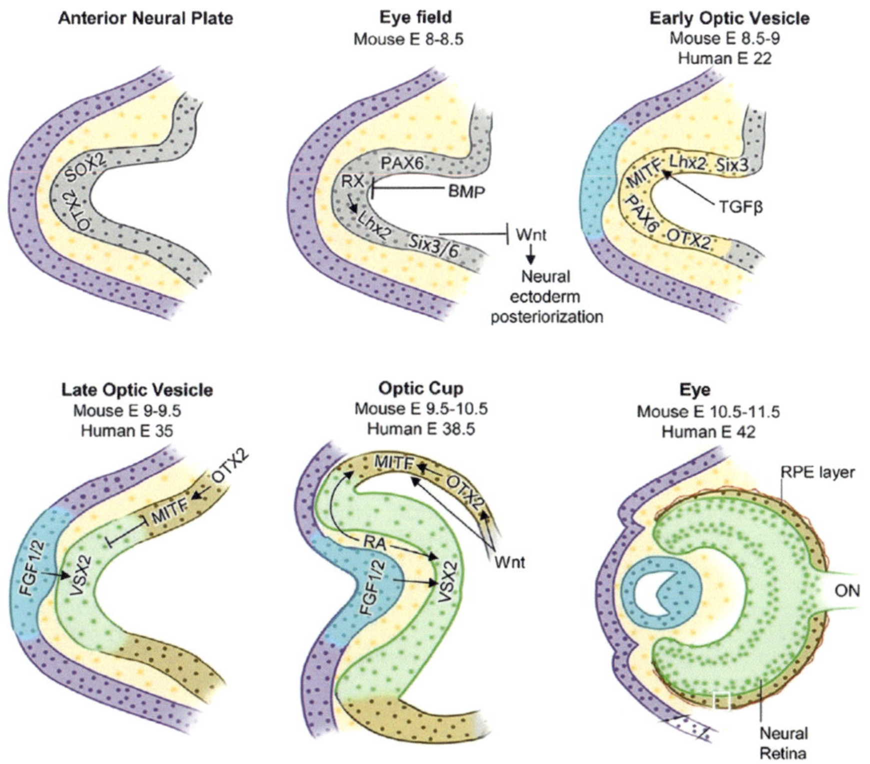

Figure 2.
Summary of the factors involved in the development of retinal cells. The protrusion of the anterior neural tube leads to the formation of the optic vesicle. Subsequently, the interaction of this ectodermal structure with the surrounding developing tissues, including the surface ectoderm, gives rise to the optic cup. A set of molecular indicators and predominant signaling pathways from the surrounding developing tissues regulate the patterning of the pigmented and neural cells of the retina [7].

advancements in the field of retinal organoids is shown in **Figure 3**. However, the foundational concepts underlying these structures can be traced back to the early 1960s and 1970s, when researchers began exploring collective cultures of retinal nerve cells. Notably, pioneering work by Stefani and Moscona in the early 1960s demonstrated that retinal cells could maintain their self-organizing capabilities under laboratory conditions [9, 18]. This discovery sparked a series of investigations into the molecular mechanisms governing the self-organization of retinal cells.

Subsequent studies revealed that environmental factors in the culture medium, such as serum and albumin, as well as the presence of specific surface proteins, play critical roles in the formation of cell aggregates at specific developmental stages [19–26]. Morphological and electron microscopy analyses of these aggregates showed the presence of rosette-like structures with central cavities, indicating a level of complexity in the organization of retinal cells [27, 28].

Advancements in cell culture techniques allowed researchers to investigate the interactions between different cell types and how they organize into more complex structures. Co-culturing RPE cells with neurons led to the formation of layered structures that more closely resembled the architecture of the native retina [29, 30].

The advent of pluripotent stem cell technology marked a significant turning point in retinal research. In 2005 and 2006, groundbreaking studies by Ikeda and

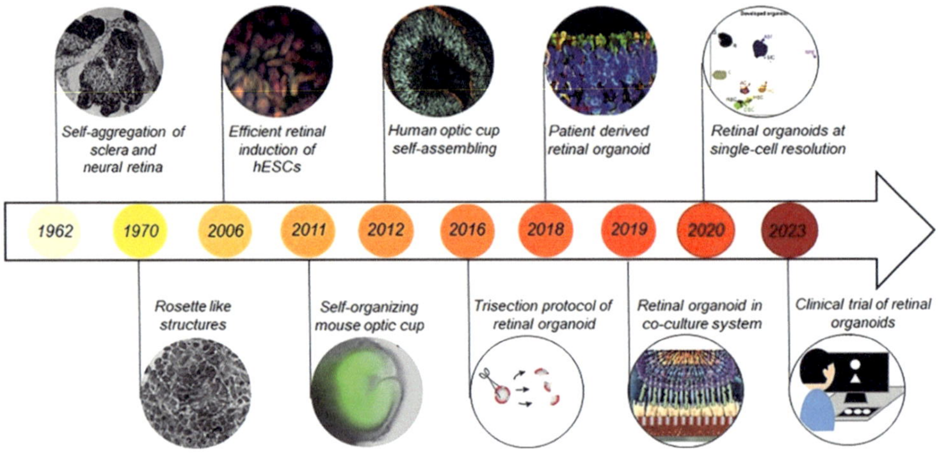

Figure 3.
Timeline of key advancements in the field of retinal organoids. 1962; self-assembly of scleral and retinal neural tissues. 1970; formation of rosette-like structures resembling the epithelial structures of neural stem cells [9]. 2006; induction of highly efficient differentiation of mouse ESCs into retinal cells [10]. 2011; self-organization of the optic cup derived from mouse ESCs [11], and in 2012; from human ESCs [12]. 2016; increased efficiency of differentiation of mouse ESCs into retinal neural cells by trisection of retinal organoid [13]. 2018; transplantation of human retinal organoids into the subretinal space of rats [14]. 2019; co-culture of retinal organoids with RPE cells and assessment of their behavior in culture [15]. 2020; evaluation of the nature of differentiated cells in retinal organoids compared to retinal cells in vivo *with single-cell resolution [16]. 2023; presentation of quality control methods and first outcome of retinal organoid transplantation in patient with retinitis pigmentosa [17].*

Lamba demonstrated the successful derivation of retinal neural progenitor cells from both mouse and human ESCs, laying the groundwork for numerous subsequent investigations [10, 31].

Recognizing the importance of 3D cell culture in mimicking natural developmental processes, Irako's team in Japan successfully generated retinal organoids from mouse ESCs in 2011 [11]. Their follow-up study in 2012 introduced the concept of "retinal self-organization," showcasing the potential of these organoids for studying retinal development [12].

By 2016, retinal organoids had gained widespread recognition, with Volkner's research demonstrating that dividing these organoids into three parts could achieve 100% differentiation of mouse ESCs into retinal organoids [13]. This breakthrough opened new avenues for modeling retinal diseases. In 2018, researchers successfully modeled retinitis pigmentosa (RP) using patient-derived iPSCs, allowing for the evaluation of molecular and developmental factors involved in the disease [14].

The functional evaluation of retinal organoids also gained traction, as demonstrated by McLand and colleagues, who transplanted retinal organoids into the subretinal space of damaged rat eyes. This approach highlighted the potential of organoids for therapeutic applications [32]. Furthermore, a 2019 study by Tasnim and colleagues found that co-culturing retinal organoids with RPE cells accelerated their differentiation, underscoring the importance of cellular interactions in organoid development [15].

In 2020, Esridhar and colleagues utilized single-cell RNA sequencing to demonstrate that organoids derived from human ESCs closely resemble the gene expression profile of the human retinal region. This finding emphasizes the relevance of retinal organoids as models for human retinal biology [16].

In the years following 2020, the field of retinal organoids has witnessed substantial progress, particularly in enhancing the maturation and functionality of these structures. A key advancement was the refinement of culture protocols, incorporating advanced technologies to mimic the natural developmental environment more closely. For example, the use of bioreactors and microfluidic systems has significantly improved the laminar stratification of retinal layers, leading to the generation of high numbers of mature photoreceptors with well-defined outer segments. Additionally, the supplementation of culture media with growth factors such as IGF1 and the use of hydrogels have accelerated the maturation of photoreceptors and enhanced their interaction with co-cultured RPE cells [33].

The period from 2020 to 2024 also saw a focus on addressing the limitations of current retinal organoid systems, such as the lack of a vascular system and batch-to-batch variability. Innovations like retinal-on-a-chip devices and assembled techniques have been explored to combine cells from different developmental lineages, thereby enhancing the morphological and functional maturation of organoids. Gene editing technologies, particularly CRISPR/Cas9, have been integrated into retinal organoid research, enabling the precise modeling of genetic retinal diseases and the evaluation of therapeutic interventions. These advancements have positioned retinal organoids as powerful tools for basic research, disease modeling, and high-throughput drug screening, paving the way for potential therapeutic applications in the treatment of retinal disorders. For instance, a 2022 study by Lee and colleagues demonstrated the successful use of CRISPR/Cas9 to correct mutations in patient-derived retinal organoids, offering new hope for gene therapy approaches. Furthermore, a 2023 study by Patel et al. showcased the potential of retinal organoids in personalized medicine by generating patient-specific models of retinal diseases, which can be used to test the efficacy of various treatments. These developments underscore the rapid progress and promising future of retinal organoid research [34–38].

Today, research in the field of retinal organoids continues to expand, with ongoing efforts aimed at enhancing the efficiency and effectiveness of generating these 3D structures. The increasing body of work highlights the potential of retinal organoids as powerful tools for understanding retinal development, disease modeling, and regenerative medicine. In 2024, Harkin established a standardized differentiation protocol that regulated the size and shape of organoids by employing rapid reaggregation techniques and precisely tuning the BMP signaling activation time in developing cells, achieving 100% efficiency across various commonly utilized cell lines [39]. The increasing body of work highlights the potential of retinal organoids as powerful tools for understanding retinal development, disease modeling, and regenerative medicine. In line with clinical application of retinal organoids, Watari reported a quality control method for tissue-sheet transplantation [40] and for the first time, safety and stable survival of retinal organoid for 2 years in patients with RP was reported [17].

3.2 Tissue-derived stem cells and their potential for organoid generation

Research on retinal organoids began with the culture of chick embryo eye cells. In these early studies, cells derived from the sclera and retina were separated from the eye and recombined. Observations revealed that the retinal and scleral cells organized into distinct groups, with the neural cells forming retinal-like structures while the scleral cells formed a dense surrounding mass [9, 18]. Utilizing spin-culture techniques, researchers were able to generate rose-like structures with a central cavity lined by ganglion cells [28].

In addition to these chick embryo studies; investigations were conducted using mammalian retinal cells. The first organotypic cultures involved separating the retinal layer from mouse tissue and maintaining it as a suspension without isolation. This culture method led to synaptic formation within the inner retinal layer [41]. Following this, Rothermel and colleagues successfully established suspension cultures of retinal cells from newborn rats, revealing the formation of distinct retinal layers over a 35-day culture period [42].

However, research in mammals was primarily limited to mice and rats, and ethical concerns surrounding the isolation of cells from larger mammals, particularly humans, posed challenges for developmental studies. The need for a reliable human cell line became increasingly apparent. Fortunately, in 1994, the first transgenic line of retinal neural progenitor cells was introduced. These cells exhibited elongated neural outgrowths and expressed specific markers characteristic of retinal neurons [43]. When cultured separately or co-cultured with RPE cells, this cell line demonstrated the ability to form 3D structures and differentiate into various retinal cell types, including photoreceptors, bipolar cells, ganglion cells, and glial cells [44, 45].

3.3 Pluripotent stem cells as a versatile source for retinal organoid development

Pluripotent stem cells (PSCs) have garnered significant attention in regenerative medicine due to their remarkable ability to proliferate and differentiate into various cell types. Unlike cells derived from tissues, PSCs are not subject to ethical limitations, making them an attractive option for research and therapeutic applications. The first successful generation of retinal structures from PSCs in a laboratory setting was reported by Sasai's group. In their pioneering study, they cultured PSCs derived from single mouse embryos in the presence of Matrigel and Nodal protein, which served as crucial factors for patterning the nervous system. Over time, these cells formed aggregates that developed into hollow spheres surrounded by a layer of epithelial cells. Gradually, protrusions resembling optic vesicles emerged from the walls of these spheres, ultimately giving rise to the optic cup [12].

In 2012, Sasai's group extended their research to human ESCs. To enhance cell survival post-isolation, they employed a Rho/ROCK pathway inhibitor. Additionally, the use of a Wnt pathway inhibitor, combined with serum reduction, significantly improved the differentiation rate of cells into anterior neural ectoderm. One week after the formation of 3D cell aggregates, structures exhibiting protrusions analogous to visual vesicles were identified, expressing the RAX transcription factor, which is critical for eye development. Continued cultivation of these structures led to the gradual formation of a two-layered optic cup. Analysis of these structures revealed the expression of specific markers, with MITF indicating RPE cells in the outer layer and CHX10 marking retinal neural progenitor cells in the inner layer. Notably, these three-dimensional structures exhibited apical-basal polarity akin to that found in living organisms.

Following the isolation of the optic cup and its suspension culture, multilayered retinal structures emerged, expressing markers characteristic of retinal nerve cells at appropriate developmental stages. During this differentiation process, cells near the basal surface exited the cell cycle, differentiated, and expressed specific markers for ganglion cells, such as BRN3a. Meanwhile, proliferation continued in the vertical axis, with the expression of Crx, a marker for photoreceptor progenitor cells, and Rcoverin, a marker for rod photoreceptors. As differentiation progressed, intermediate cells also exhibited markers for bipolar cells (CHX10), horizontal cells (Calbindin), and amacrine cells (Calretinin).

Despite these advancements in the 3D culture of retinal cells, challenges remained, particularly regarding size limitations due to diffusion constraints for gases and nutrients within the organoids. This led to studies exploring the combination of 2D and 3D culture techniques [46–49]. In this approach, cells were mechanically processed to form embryo-like bodies, which were then cultured in suspension and induced toward neural ectoderm. Subsequent culture on a Matrigel-covered substrate allowed for the differentiation of neural and non-neural retinal layers. The resulting tube-like structures were isolated from the substrate and further characterized as retinal organoids, displaying distinct pigmented areas and neural epithelium.

In some studies, researchers opted for high-density cultures of pluripotent stem cells instead of starting with embryonic-like bodies. This dense culture environment promotes the release of Wnt pathway inhibitors, such as DKK, which guide cells toward an anterior neural fate, eliminating the need for external inhibitors.

In 2021, Vagsteff and colleagues reviewed various studies and identified that the lack of uniformity in retinal organoid production is often linked to the use of different activators or inhibitors of cellular signaling pathways. They noted that the effects of these pathways can be synergistic, further complicating the differentiation process [50]. To address this variability, a novel approach involves fragmenting retinal organoids after the formation of visual vesicles. By using a glass pipette, the organoids can be divided into smaller pieces, which are then cultured in conditions conducive to the maturation of precursor cells into photoreceptors. This method not only enhances the expression of eye-specific markers but also allows for better nutrient diffusion and expansion, resulting in a larger yield of retinal organoids while preserving the layered structure of the retina [51].

Additionally, to extend the culture period of these organoids up to 60 days, researchers enriched the culture medium with Shh pathway agonists at various intervals. This strategy promoted continued cell development, resulting in the presence of all major retinal cell types within the layered structure. By prolonging the culture conditions, researchers aim to increase the number of required cells and create a model for studying various pathological retinal malformations, thereby enhancing the potential applications of retinal organoids in both research and therapeutic contexts [52].

By refining culture conditions and leveraging the versatility of PSCss, researchers can continue to advance our understanding of retinal development and explore the potential applications of these organoids in regenerative medicine and disease modeling.

4. Engineering strategies for retinal organoids

4.1 Dynamic culture systems and biomimetic scaffolds and their role in recapitulating the native retinal niche

While traditional 2D culture methods are widely used due to their simplicity and accessibility, 3D culture systems have gained significant interest among researchers. This shift is largely attributed to the enhanced importance of cell interactions and the closer resemblance to the physiological conditions of living organisms. Despite the advantages of 3D models, they still encounter several limitations, which can be addressed through various bioengineering strategies.

One of the primary challenges in 3D retinal organoid cultures is ensuring that nutrients effectively reach the innermost cells of the organoid. To overcome this issue, rotating flasks and dynamic culture systems have been proposed to facilitate nutrient distribution. The limitations associated with nutrient and oxygen diffusion in 3D cultures highlight the advantages of bioreactor systems over static cultures.

Additionally, other limitations include inadequate cell interactions on the organoid surface and the absence of a suitable coating that mimics lens induction during development. Matrigel has been commonly utilized in numerous studies to provide a supportive matrix; however, recent engineering approaches have suggested the use of various hydrogels to optimize retinal organoid cultivation. These hydrogels aim to enhance the formation of visual vesicles and support their differentiation into optic cups. For instance, a study demonstrated that encapsulating retinal organoids in an alginate hydrogel modified with the arginine-glycine-aspartic acid (RGD) peptide significantly improved cell survival and increased the efficiency of visual vesicle formation, as well as the continued production of the RPE cells these culture conditions.

The specific interactions facilitated by biomimetic scaffolds are essential for recapitulating the native retinal niche, ultimately contributing to improved outcomes in retinal tissue engineering and regenerative medicine.

4.2 Specialized chip and bioprinting technology optimization to support retinal organoid maturation

In the realm of retinal organoid culture, innovative approaches such as bioprinting and the optimization of extracellular matrices (ECMs) are pivotal for enhancing organoid maturation. A notable study employed the Cellfoil chip for 3D cell culture, which is constructed from polymethyl methacrylate (PMMA) and features a perforated polycarbonate plate. This chip houses 506 microcontainers, each measuring $300 \times 300 \times 300$ micrometers, capable of accommodating approximately 6×10^6 cells. The chip is integrated into a bioreactor equipped with a closed circulation system, a pump, and a source of culture medium connected to a gas mixing tank. Utilizing this setup, over 80% of spheroids formed with uniform shapes, and retinal organoid-specific markers were expressed similarly to those in rotary culture models. Notably, the cells derived from this culture exhibited differentiation into amacrine cells and their neural projections within the organoid's internal space, resembling the inner retinal layers [53].

The field of retinal tissue engineering has seen significant advancements using bioprinting techniques for the 3D simulation of retinal tissues and organs in a laboratory setting. Hydrogels have emerged as a versatile bioink for the 3D reconstruction of retinal tissue structures. While natural hydrogels may not possess the necessary strength to form a robust gel with cells in their native state, chemical modifications can enhance their properties. By introducing light-sensitive functional groups, such as methacrylates, hydrogels can be polymerized upon exposure to light, improving their physicochemical properties and making them suitable for cell printing applications [54].

Another bioprinting approach utilizes rapid ink release to preserve the differentiation of mature photoreceptor cells derived from porcine eyes, co-cultured with ARPE-19 retinal pigment cells. Photoreceptor cells printed using this layered system maintained the expression of their differentiation markers at the protein level even 1 week after printing [55].

These advancements in bioprinting technology have significantly contributed to the field of retinal tissue engineering, allowing for the precise and controlled fabrication of complex retinal tissue structures that closely mimic the native retinal microenvironment. The ability to print multiple cell types in a layered arrangement and maintain their differentiation status highlights the potential of bioprinting in regenerative medicine applications targeting retinal diseases and disorders.

5. Retinal organoids in disease and therapy

3D retinal organoids, derived from the self-organization of ESCs or iPSCs, exhibit cellular and functional characteristics akin to those of the native retina. This resemblance makes retinal organoids an invaluable tool for investigating the molecular mechanisms underlying various eye diseases, screening potential therapeutic agents, and exploring cell therapy options. The extensive applications of these organoids in disease modeling and therapeutic development are outlined below [56].

Retinal organoids provide a unique human model system that allows researchers to study the pathogenesis of retinal diseases and to develop new therapeutic strategies. Their ability to mimic the structural and functional aspects of the retina facilitates the exploration of disease mechanisms and the evaluation of drug efficacy in a more physiologically relevant context than traditional 2D models [56].

Recent advancements in retinal organoid technology have enabled high-throughput screening of small molecules, which is crucial for identifying potential treatments for various retinal disorders. This approach has been successfully applied to discover candidate drugs and assess their effects on retinal cell differentiation and function. Furthermore, retinal organoids derived from patient-specific iPSCs allow for personalized medicine approaches, providing insights into individual disease phenotypes and responses to therapy [56].

Despite the promising potential of retinal organoids, several challenges remain. For instance, while these organoids can model certain aspects of retinal diseases, they often exhibit limited functionality, such as poor light responsiveness, due to the absence of direct interactions with RPE cells and other supporting structures. Additionally, the variability in maturation states and the heterogeneity of cell types within organoids can complicate comparative analyses and therapeutic assessments [56]. To address these limitations, researchers are exploring innovative strategies, such as co-culturing retinal organoids with RPE cells or integrating organoid systems with organ-on-a-chip technologies. These approaches aim to enhance the maturity and functionality of retinal organoids, thereby improving their utility in drug discovery and disease modeling [56].

In summary, retinal organoids represent a powerful platform for understanding retinal diseases and developing novel therapies. Their ability to recapitulate key features of the human retina positions them as a critical resource in the pursuit of effective treatments for retinal disorders, ultimately advancing the field of regenerative medicine.

5.1 Leveraging retinal organoids for disease modeling and mechanistic studies

Retinal diseases and syndromes often lead to vision loss, underscoring the urgent need for effective treatments. Animal models, such as dogs, cats, chickens, pigs, and rodents, have been instrumental in evaluating various aspects of the retina. However, the human eye is unique in several ways, including the macula and the complexity of color perception. As a result, not all diseases and drug responses can be fully replicated in animal models. There is a pressing need for systems that incorporate both genetic background and anatomical and cellular phenomena [56].

Inherited retinal diseases (IRDs) are a category of genetic disorders marked by progressive vision loss resulting from the degeneration of retinal cells. These diseases present a diverse array of clinical characteristics, including variations in onset, symptoms, progression, and severity. IRDs can occur at various stages of life, from early childhood to later adulthood, and may be classified as non-syndromic (affecting only the retina) or syndromic (involving other organs). The genetic complexity and diversity of IRDs, with over 260 implicated genes, pose significant challenges for diagnosis and research. Current treatment strategies primarily focus on gene therapy, such as the FDA-approved Luxturna for RPE65-related dystrophy, alongside experimental approaches like CRISPR/Cas9 for other IRDs, and cell therapies aimed at replacing lost photoreceptors, providing hope for patients with advanced IRDs [57].

In this context, the advent of iPSCs technology enables the generation of pluripotent stem cells from individuals with genetic diseases. By creating disease models from these patient-derived cells, researchers can perform drug screening and assess the developmental impacts of genetic disorders [56].

One study found that disruption of the USH2A gene, a major cause of RP, leads to the formation of misfolded proteins and endoplasmic reticulum stress. Additionally, organoids with USH2A mutations show decreased laminin expression and impaired development of retinal pigment cells, cilia, and dopaminergic synapses. Conversely, genes involved in apoptotic cell death are upregulated [56, 58].

Leber congenital amaurosis (LCA) is a severe childhood vision disorder that can lead to blindness. Fourteen candidate genes have been identified for LCA, with many mutations located in cilia-related genes [59]. By using iPSCs derived from LCA patients with specific gene mutations, researchers can model the disease in retinal organoids. One study focused on the CEP290 gene, which encodes a centrosomal ciliary protein. Retinal organoids derived from CEP290-mutant iPSCs exhibited impaired ciliogenesis, which was partially restored by treatment with CEP290 antisense morpholino [14].

Retinal organoids have also been used to model other vision disorders, such as microphthalmia, a developmental disorder characterized by abnormally small eye size and anatomical disturbances. By disrupting the VSX2 gene, researchers created a microphthalmia model in organoids and evaluated the transcription factors and signaling pathways involved [60].

Glaucoma, a prevalent disorder characterized by ganglion cell defects, arises from a combination of genetic and environmental factors. Retinal organoids have been utilized to model hereditary glaucoma associated with mutations in the optineurin gene (OPTN) [61].

Retinoblastoma, a childhood cancer that develops during retinal formation, is characterized by the bilateral inactivation of the RB1 gene. To model this disease, researchers generated a series of iPSC lines from individuals with this genetic defect. These cells were subsequently differentiated into retinal organoids *in vitro* [62].

Recent studies utilizing these laboratory models have demonstrated significant progress in retinal disease regeneration, leveraging patient-derived cells to address various retinal cell damage scenarios. Consequently, retinal organoids serve as valuable models for investigating retinal cell disorders, aiding in the understanding of the molecular mechanisms that drive these diseases and facilitating the development of targeted treatment solutions, in this regards some studies reviewed in more details in **Table 1**.

Retinal diseases	Associated genes	Type of mutation	Primary affected cells	Reprogramming methods	Phenotypic changes and cellular outcomes	Ref.
Normal tension glaucoma	*OPTN*	E50K	Fibroblast	mRNA (OKSM*)	The Golgi apparatus in iPSCs with OPTN mutation exhibits disorganized morphology leading to an increase in cell size. Caspase 3 activity is elevated in ganglion cells derived from these cells. The treatment of these ganglion cells with the growth factors BDNF and PEDF result in partial rescue from apoptosis.	[63]
Dominant optic atrophy	*OPA1*	Intron24 c.2496 + 1 G > T	Fibroblast	Retrovirus (OKSM)	Apoptosis was significantly increased in iPSCs with OPA1 mutation. The presence of Noggin or estrogen enhance the differentiation efficiency of OPT-1 mutated iPSCs into ganglion cells.	[64]
Leber's hereditary optic neuropathy (LHON)	*MIND1* *MIND4*	m.4160 T > C and m.14,484 T > C	Fibroblast	Episomal (Lin28/ OKSM/shRNAp53)	The production of isogenic iPSCs was controlled by replacing the mitochondrial DNA of a patient with LHON using cybrid technology. This approach allowed for the observation of changes in apoptosis level in ganglion cells derived from the LHON patients iPSCs.	[65]

The four transcription factors OCT4, KLF4, SOX2, and MYC (OKSM) together can convert human fibroblasts to induced pluripotent stem cells (iPSCs).

Table 1.
Some studies on retinal organoids for investigating the molecular mechanisms that drive these diseases.

These findings underscore the utility of retinal organoids in elucidating the effects of genetic mutations on retinal integrity and functionality, paving the way for novel therapeutic strategies and a deeper understanding of retinal diseases.

5.2 Retinal organoids in drug screening, discovery, and regeneration

Retinal degenerative diseases pose significant challenges, affecting millions worldwide. Recent estimates indicate that approximately 8.5 million people suffer from age-related macular degeneration, 4 million from glaucoma, and 2.5 million from diabetic retinopathy. The individual and economic impact of these conditions is profound, highlighting the urgent need for effective treatments [66]. Despite advancements in reconstruction technologies, many of these innovations have yet to translate into clinical applications, leaving patients reliant on traditional methods to manage or prevent disease progression. Alarmingly, since 2015, only 13.8% of drugs have successfully navigated the approval process from initial clinical trials to final approval, with the average cost for bringing a drug to market reaching around $5 billion [67].

One of the major obstacles in developing new therapies is the lack of reliable evaluation methods within drug production lines. However, the advent of 3D retinal organoids presents a promising opportunity to enhance or replace traditional drug evaluation methods.

Given these advancements, retinal organoids serve as a powerful intermediary between 2D cultures and animal models, allowing for more accurate drug screening and reducing unnecessary animal costs. The scientific community is increasingly focused on translating basic research into clinical applications. The integration of drug screening with disease modeling holds great promise for advancing precision medicine applications in the future.

5.3 Exploring the use of retinal organoids in developmental biology research

Recent advancements in differentiation techniques have enabled the generation of retinal organoids that closely resemble retinal cells in an extracorporeal environment. As a result, researchers have increasingly turned to retinal organoids to investigate the molecular events involved in retinal development, moving away from traditional *in vivo* studies. For instance, a study by Gabriel and colleagues demonstrated that visual vesicles begin to form bilaterally 30 days after the establishment of brain organoids, with this process continuing until the 60th day of differentiation. These visual vesicles exhibit many properties characteristic of native structures, including corneal epithelium, lens-like cells, RPE cells, retinal progenitor cells, axonal outgrowths, and electrically active neural retinas [68].

During retinal histogenesis, retinal progenitor cells differentiate into various types of retinal neurons at specific times and locations. Notably, cylindrical photoreceptor cells emerge in the later stages of development, outnumbering cone photoreceptor cells significantly [69].

These findings underscore the potential of retinal organoids as a powerful model for studying developmental biology, offering insights into the molecular mechanisms underlying retinal development and providing a platform for future research into retinal diseases and regenerative therapies.

DOI: http://dx.doi.org/10.5772/intechopen.1007790

5.4 Advancements in retinal organoid-based regenerative medicine approaches

The development of 3D retinal organoids has significantly enhanced their application in regenerative medicine. A primary objective of research in this field is to identify reliable cell types or populations that can be effectively transplanted into the eye. Studies have demonstrated that retinal neural progenitor cells are particularly suitable for transplantation into the ocular space of animal models with damaged neural cells, making cell therapy a promising solution.

The conditions under which cells are transferred—whether in suspension or as 3D structures—are crucial for successful integration. In some studies, ESCs are first differentiated into retinal organoids, from which goblet structures are isolated through enzymatic digestion before being transplanted into the ocular space of disease models [70]. To enrich the transferred cell populations and ensure their efficacy, specific surface biomarkers are used for isolation and monitoring. One such biomarker is CD73, which indicates a lower likelihood of tumorigenesis, as cells expressing CD73 do not also express the proliferative marker Ki67 [69].

Transplanting retinal organoids as 3D structures represents another innovative approach in regenerative medicine. After deriving retinal organoids from ESCs, these organoid structures can be directly transferred to the subretinal space of animal models [71, 72].

Despite the significant progress made, challenges remain, particularly concerning the compatibility of donor and recipient cell types during transplantation and stronger and more direct evidence is required to fully evaluate the potential of retinal organoids in cell therapy studies.

6. Conclusion and future perspectives

The advent of organoid technology has revolutionized laboratory research, bridging significant gaps in developmental and medical biology. As discussed throughout this chapter, substantial progress has been made in the generation of retinal organoids. By utilizing iPSCs, researchers can obtain stem cells with specific gene mutations from affected individuals and differentiate these cells into organoids to investigate the molecular mechanisms underlying retinal diseases. This laboratory model not only facilitates the examination of disease formation but also enables the screening of various compounds proposed as potential preclinical drugs. Ultimately, the goal is to develop complex retinal organoids that closely resemble native retinal structures, paving the way for advancements in organ transplantation and regenerative medicine.

Despite these promising developments, challenges remain in optimizing retinal organoid culture conditions, necessitating further efforts to standardize long-term culture protocols. One significant issue is the immaturity of photoreceptor cell outer segments in the resulting organoids. The lack of interaction with RPE cells may contribute to this immaturity, as studies have indicated that dysfunctional RPE cells are associated with impaired morphogenesis of photoreceptor outer segments [73].

Additionally, the morphological and functional variability among different cell lines presents another challenge in organoid production. Variations in differentiation methods and the timing of neural cell development must be thoroughly investigated to enhance consistency and reliability.

To effectively translate these findings into clinical applications, it is essential to establish standardized protocols for generating retinal organoids and to conduct large-scale evaluations. With ongoing research and advancements in this field, there is optimism that these goals can be achieved soon, ultimately leading to improved therapies for retinal degenerative diseases.

Acknowledgements

We would like to thank Miss Elahe sadat Mirsane for preparing the figures. We apologize to all authors whose works have not been included or adequately discussed because of space limitations. This work was supported by Royan Institute.

Conflict of interest

The authors declare that they have no competing interests.

Author details

Reyhaneh Sadat Mousavi[1], Fatemeh Naghshnejad[1], Fereshteh Karamali[2] and Leila Satarian[3*]

1 Royan Institute, Tehran, Iran

2 Royan Institute, Isfahan, Iran

3 Department of Stem Cells and Developmental Biology, Cell Science Research Center, Royan Institute for Stem Cell Biology and Technology, ACECR, Tehran, Iran

*Address all correspondence to: l.satarian@royan-rc.ac.ir

References

[1] Pearson RA, Barber A, Rizzi M, Hippert C, Xue T, West E, et al. Restoration of vision after transplantation of photoreceptors. Nature. 2012;**485**(7396):99-103

[2] Singh MS, Charbel Issa P, Butler R, Martin C, Lipinski DM, Sekaran S, et al. Reversal of end-stage retinal degeneration and restoration of visual function by photoreceptor transplantation. National Academy of Sciences of the United States of America. 2013;**110**(3):1101-1106

[3] Ortin-Martinez A, Tsai ELS, Nickerson PE, Bergeret M, Lu Y, Smiley S, et al. A reinterpretation of cell transplantation: GFP transfer from donor to host photoreceptors. Stem Cells. 2017;**35**(4):932-939

[4] Willoughby CE, Ponzin D, Ferrari S, Lobo A, Landau K, Omidi Y. Anatomy and physiology of the human eye: Effects of mucopolysaccharidoses disease on structure and function—A review. Clinical and Experimental Ophthalmology. 2010;**38**:2-11

[5] Strauss O. The retinal pigment epithelium in visual function. Physiological Reviews; 1 Jul 2005

[6] Stern CD. Neural induction: 10 years on since the 'default model'. Current Opinion in Cell Biology. 2006;**18**(6):692-697

[7] Parvini M, Satarian L, Parivar K, Javan M, Tondar M, Ahmad S, et al. Human pluripotent stem cell-derived retinal pigmented epithelium in retinal treatment: From bench to bedside. Molecular Neurobiology. 2014;**50**(2):597-612

[8] Volkner M, Zschatzsch M, Rostovskaya M, Overall RW, Busskamp V, Anastassiadis K, et al. Retinal organoids from pluripotent stem cells efficiently recapitulate retinogenesis. Stem Cell Reports. 2016;**6**(4):525-538

[9] Lilien JE, Moscona A. Cell aggregation: Its enhancement by a supernatant from cultures of homologous cells. Science. 1967;**157**(3784):70-72

[10] Lamba DA, Karl MO, Ware CB, Reh TA. Efficient generation of retinal progenitor cells from human embryonic stem cells. National Academy of Sciences of the United States of America. 2006;**103**(34):12769-12774

[11] Eiraku M, Takata N, Ishibashi H, Kawada M, Sakakura E, Okuda S, et al. Self-organizing optic-cup morphogenesis in three-dimensional culture. Nature. 2011;**472**(7341):51-56

[12] Nakano T, Ando S, Takata N, Kawada M, Muguruma K, Sekiguchi K, et al. Self-formation of optic cups and storablestratifiedneuralretinafromhuman ESCs. Cell Stem Cell. 2012;**10**(6):771-785

[13] Parfitt DA, Lane A, Ramsden CM, Carr A-JF, Munro PM, Jovanovic K, et al. Identification and correction of mechanisms underlying inherited blindness in human iPSC-derived optic cups. Cell Stem Cell. 2016;**18**(6):769-781

[14] McLelland BT, Lin B, Mathur A, Aramant RB, Thomas BB, Nistor G, et al. Transplanted hESC-derived retina organoid sheets differentiate, integrate, and improve visual function in retinal degenerate rats. Investigative Ophthalmology and Visual Science. 2018;**59**(6):2586-2603

[15] Sridhar A, Hoshino A, Finkbeiner CR, Chitsazan A,

Dai L, Haugan AK, et al. Single-cell transcriptomic comparison of human fetal retina, hPSC-derived retinal organoids, and long-term retinal cultures. Cell Reports. 2020;**30**(5): 1644-59.e4

[16] Bytyqi AH, Bachmann G, Rieke M, Paraoanu LE, Layer PG. Cell-by-cell reconstruction in reaggregates from neonatal gerbil retina begins from the inner retina and is promoted by retinal pigmented epithelium. European Journal of Neuroscience. 2007;**26**(6):1560-1574

[17] Hirami Y, Mandai M, Sugita S, Maeda A, Maeda T, Yamamoto M, et al. Safety and stable survival of stem-cell-derived retinal organoid for 2 years in patients with retinitis pigmentosa. Cell Stem Cell. 2023;**30**(12):1585-96.e6

[18] Stefanelli A, Zacchei A, Ceccherini V. Retinal reconstitution in vitro after disaggregation of embryonic chicken eyes (translated from Italian). Acta Embryologiae et Morphologiae Experimentalis. 1961;**4**:47-55

[19] Richmond JE, Glaeser RM. Effect of culture media on self-organization and protein synthesis of neural retina cells. Comparative Biochemistry and Physiology Part B: Comparative Biochemistry. 1971;**40**(2):327-334

[20] Armstrong PB. A fine structural study of adhesive cell junctions in heterotypic cell aggregates. The Journal of Cell Biology. 1970;**47**(1):197

[21] Daday H. The mechanism of aggregation of neural retina cells in vitro. Wilhelm Roux' Archiv für Entwicklungsmechanik der Organismen. 1972;**171**(3):244-255

[22] Geller RL, Lilien J. Repair of a calcium-dependent adhesive mechanism of embryonic neural retina cells: Kinetic and molecular analysis. Journal of Cell Science. 1983;**60**(1):29-49

[23] Matsunaga M, Hatta K, Takeichi M. Role of N-cadherin cell adhesion molecules in the histogenesis of neural retina. Neuron. 1988;**1**(4):289-295

[24] Orr CW, Roseman S. Intercellular adhesion: II. The purification and properties of a horse serum protein that promotes neural retina cell aggregation. The Journal of Membrane Biology. 1969;**1**:125-143

[25] Thomas WA, Steinberg MS. Two distinct adhesion mechanisms in embryonic neural retina cells: II. An immunological analysis. Developmental Biology. 1981;**81**(1):106-114

[26] Sheffield JB, Moscona A. Electron microscopic analysis of aggregation of embryonic cells: The structure and differentiation of aggregates of neural retina cells. Developmental Biology. 1970;**23**(1):36-61

[27] Fujisawa H. The process of reconstruction of histological architecture from dissociated retinal cells. Wilhelm Roux' Archiv für Entwicklungsmechanik der Organismen. 1973;**171**(4):312-330

[28] Rothermel A, Willbold E, Degrip WJ, Layer PG. Pigmented epithelium induces complete retinal reconstitution from dispersed embryonic chick retinae in reaggregation culture. Proceedings of the Royal Society of London, Series B: Biological Sciences. 1997;**264**(1386):1293-1302

[29] Vollmer G, Layer P, Gierer A. Reaggregation of embryonic chick retina cells: Pigment epithelial cells induce a high order of stratification. Neuroscience Letters. 1984;**48**(2):191-196

[30] Armstrong PB. Light and electron microscope studies of cell sorting in combinations of chick embryo neural retina and retinal pigment epithelium. Wilhelm Roux' Archiv für Entwicklungsmechanik der Organismen. 1971;**168**:125-141

[31] Ikeda H, Osakada F, Watanabe K, Mizuseki K, Haraguchi T, Miyoshi H, et al. Generation of Rx+/Pax6+ neural retinal precursors from embryonic stem cells. National Academy of Sciences of the United States of America. 2005;**102**(32):11331-11336

[32] Akhtar T, Xie H, Khan MI, Zhao H, Bao J, Zhang M, et al. Accelerated photoreceptor differentiation of hiPSC-derived retinal organoids by contact co-culture with retinal pigment epithelium. Stem Cell Research. 2019;**39**:101491

[33] Sharma K, Krohne TU, Busskamp V. The rise of retinal organoids for vision research. International Journal of Molecular Sciences. 11 Nov 2020;**21**(22):8484

[34] O'Hara-Wright M, Gonzalez-Cordero A. Retinal organoids: a window into human retinal development. Development. 15 Dec 2020;**147**(24):dev189746

[35] Afanasyeva TAV, Corral-Serrano JC, Garanto A, Roepman R, Cheetham ME, Collin RWJ. A look into retinal organoids: Methods, analytical techniques, and applications. Cellular and Molecular Life Sciences. 2021;**78**(19-20):6505-6532

[36] Bellapianta A, Cetkovic A, Bolz M, Salti A. Retinal organoids and retinal prostheses: an overview. International journal of molecular sciences. 8 Mar 2022;**23**(6):2922

[37] Ovando-Roche P, West EL, Branch MJ, Sampson RD, Fernando M, Munro P, et al. Use of bioreactors for culturing human retinal organoids improves photoreceptor yields. Stem Cell Research & Therapy. 2018;**9**(1):156

[38] Li X, Zhang L, Tang F, Wei X. Retinal organoids: Cultivation, differentiation, and transplantation. Frontiers in Cellular Neuroscience. 2021;**15**:638439

[39] Harkin J, Peña KH, Gomes C, Hernandez M, Lavekar SS, So K, et al. A highly reproducible and efficient method for retinal organoid differentiation from human pluripotent stem cells. National Academy of Sciences of the United States of America. 2024;**121**(25):e2317285121

[40] Watari K, Yamasaki S, Tu HY, Shikamura M, Kamei T, Adachi H, et al. Self-organization, quality control, and preclinical studies of human iPSC-derived retinal sheets for tissue-transplantation therapy. Communications Biology. 2023;**6**(1):164

[41] Rothermel A, Biedermann T, Weigel W, Kurz R, Rüffer M, Layer PG, et al. Artificial design of three-dimensional retina-like tissue from dissociated cells of the mammalian retina by rotation-mediated cell aggregation. Tissue Engineering. 2005;**11**(11-12):1749-1756

[42] Dutt K, Scott M, Wang M, Semple E, Sharma GP, Srinivasan A. Establishment of a human retinal cell line by transfection of SV40 T antigen gene with potential to undergo neuronal differentiation. DNA and Cell Biology. 1994;**13**(9):909-921

[43] Dutt K, Cao Y. Engineering retina from human retinal progenitors (cell lines). Tissue Engineering Parts A. 2009;**15**(6):1401-1413

[44] Gamm DM, Wright LS, Capowski EE, Shearer RL, Meyer JS, Kim H-J, et al. Regulation of prenatal

human retinal neurosphere growth and cell fate potential by retinal pigment epithelium and Mash1. Stem Cells. 2008;**26**(12):3182-3193

[45] Meyer JS, Shearer RL, Capowski EE, Wright LS, Wallace KA, McMillan EL, et al. Modeling early retinal development with human embryonic and induced pluripotent stem cells. National Academy of Sciences of the United States of America. 2009;**106**(39):16698-16703

[46] Zhong X, Gutierrez C, Xue T, Hampton C, Vergara MN, Cao L-H, et al. Generation of three-dimensional retinal tissue with functional photoreceptors from human iPSCs. Nature Communications. 2014;**5**(1):4047

[47] Gonzalez-Cordero A, Kruczek K, Naeem A, Fernando M, Kloc M, Ribeiro J, et al. Recapitulation of human retinal development from human pluripotent stem cells generates transplantable populations of cone photoreceptors. Stem Cell Reports. 2017;**9**(3):820-837

[48] Capowski EE, Samimi K, Mayerl SJ, Phillips MJ, Pinilla I, Howden SE, et al. Reproducibility and staging of 3D human retinal organoids across multiple pluripotent stem cell lines. Development. 2019;**146**(1):dev171686

[49] Reichman S, Terray A, Slembrouck A, Nanteau C, Orieux G, Habeler W, et al. From confluent human iPS cells to self-forming neural retina and retinal pigmented epithelium. National Academy of Sciences of the United States of America. 2014;**111**(23):8518-8523

[50] Wagstaff EL, Heredero Berzal A, Boon CJ, Quinn PM, Ten Asbroek AL, Bergen AA. The role of small molecules and their effect on the molecular mechanisms of early retinal organoid development. International Journal of Molecular Sciences. 2021;**22**(13):7081

[51] Moscona AA. Analysis of cell recombinations in experimental synthesis of tissues in vitro. Journal of Cellular and Comparative Physiology. 1962;**60**(S1):65-80

[52] Völkner M, Kurth T, Schor J, Ebner LJ, Bardtke L, Kavak C, et al. Mouse retinal organoid growth and maintenance in longer-term culture. Frontiers in Cell and Developmental Biology. 2021;**9**:645704

[53] Achberger K, Probst C, Haderspeck J, Bolz S, Rogal J, Chuchuy J, et al. Merging organoid and organ-on-a-chip technology to generate complex multi-layer tissue models in a human retina-on-a-chip platform. eLife. 2019;**8**:e46188

[54] Agmon G, Christman KL. Controlling stem cell behavior with decellularized extracellular matrix scaffolds. Current Opinion in Solid State and Materials Science. 2016;**20**(4):193-201

[55] Burdick JA, Prestwich GD. Hyaluronic acid hydrogels for biomedical applications. Advanced Materials. 2011;**23**(12):H41-H56

[56] Shi P, Tan YSE, Yeong WY, Li HY, Laude A. A bilayer photoreceptor-retinal tissue model with gradient cell density design: A study of microvalve-based bioprinting. Journal of Tissue Engineering and Regenerative Medicine. 2018;**12**(5):1297-1306

[57] Ashworth KE, Weisbrod J, Ballios BG. Inherited retinal diseases and retinal organoids as preclinical cell models for inherited retinal disease research. Genes. 2024;**15**(6):705

[58] Artero Castro A, Rodríguez Jimenez FJ, Jendelova P, Erceg S. Deciphering retinal diseases through the generation of three dimensional stem cell-derived organoids: Concise review. Stem Cells. 2019;**37**(12):1496-1504

[59] Arno G, Agrawal SA, Eblimit A, Bellingham J, Xu M, Wang F, et al. Mutations in REEP6 cause autosomal-recessive retinitis pigmentosa. The American Journal of Human Genetics. 2016;**99**(6):1305-1315

[60] Bavelloni A, Piazzi M, Raffini M, Faenza I, Blalock WL. Prohibitin 2: At a communications crossroads. IUBMB Life. 2015;**67**(4):239-254

[61] Bohrer LR, Wiley LA, Burnight ER, Cooke JA, Giacalone JC, Anfinson KR, et al. Correction of NR2E3 associated enhanced S-cone syndrome patient-specific iPSCs using CRISPR-Cas9. Genes. 2019;**10**(4):278

[62] Norrie JL, Nityanandam A, Lai K, Chen X, Wilson M, Stewart E, et al. Retinoblastoma from human stem cell-derived retinal organoids. Nature Communications. 2021;**12**(1):4535

[63] Ohlemacher SK, Sridhar A, Xiao Y, Hochstetler AE, Sarfarazi M, Cummins TR, et al. Stepwise differentiation of retinal ganglion cells from human pluripotent stem cells enables analysis of glaucomatous neurodegeneration. Stem Cells. 2016;**34**(6):1553-1562

[64] Chen J, Riazifar H, Guan M-X, Huang T. Modeling autosomal dominant optic atrophy using induced pluripotent stem cells and identifying potential therapeutic targets. Stem Cell Research & Therapy. 2016;**7**:1-14

[65] Wong RC, Lim SY, Hung SS, Jackson S, Khan S, Van Bergen NJ, et al. Mitochondrial replacement in an iPSC model of Leber's hereditary optic neuropathy. Aging (Albany NY). 2017;**9**(4):1341

[66] Bolinches-Amorós A, Lukovic D, Castro AA, León M, Kamenarova K, Kaneva R, et al. Generation of a human iPSC line from a patient with congenital glaucoma caused by mutation in CYP1B1 gene. Stem Cell Research. 2018;**28**:96-99

[67] Wong CH, Siah KW, Lo AW. Estimation of clinical trial success rates and related parameters. Biostatistics. 2019;**20**(2):273-286

[68] Gabriel E, Albanna W, Pasquini G, Ramani A, Josipovic N, Mariappan A, et al. Human brain organoids assemble functionally integrated bilateral optic vesicles. Cell Stem Cell. 2021;**28**(10):1740-1757 e8

[69] Kautzmann M-AI, Kim DS, Felder-Schmittbuhl M-P, Swaroop A. Combinatorial regulation of photoreceptor differentiation factor, neural retina leucine zipper gene NRL, revealed by in vivo promoter analysis. Journal of Biological Chemistry. 2011;**286**(32):28247-28255

[70] Aasen DM, Vergara MN. New drug discovery paradigms for retinal diseases: A focus on retinal organoids. Journal of Ocular Pharmacology and Therapeutics. 2020;**36**(1):18-24

[71] Zou T, Gao L, Zeng Y, Li Q, Li Y, Chen S, et al. Organoid-derived C-Kit+/SSEA4− human retinal progenitor cells promote a protective retinal microenvironment during transplantation in rodents. Nature Communications. 2019;**10**(1):1205

[72] Collin J, Zerti D, Queen R, Santos-Ferreira T, Bauer R, Coxhead J, et al. CRX expression in pluripotent stem cell-derived photoreceptors marks a transplantable subpopulation of early cones. Stem Cells. 2019;**37**(5):609-622

[73] Veleri S, Lazar CH, Chang B, Sieving PA, Banin E, Swaroop A. Biology and therapy of inherited retinal degenerative disease: Insights from mouse models. Disease Models and Mechanisms. 2015;**8**(2):109-129

Chapter 4

X-Linked Retinitis Pigmentosa Gene Therapy: Preclinical Aspects

Vahid Mansouri and Maryam Bemanalizadeh

Abstract

Retinitis pigmentosa (RP) is the most common hereditary retinal disease, with X-linked RP (XLRP) being one of the most severe forms. Individuals with XLRP progressively lose their vision, often becoming blind by their fourth decade of life, leading to significant morbidity. Currently, treatments for XLRP are insufficient to restore vision. However, gene therapy targeting the Retinitis Pigmentosa GTPase Regulator (RPGR) gene has shown encouraging results in preclinical studies and clinical trials, although no approved therapy has reached the market yet. The development of such treatments necessitates rigorous preclinical testing in animal models before being applied to humans. This review examines the genetic basis of XLRP, discusses the preclinical aspects of gene therapy in animal models, and explores future challenges and directions.

Keywords: retinitis pigmentosa, gene therapy, adeno-associated virus, retinitis pigmentosa GTPase regulator (RPGR), preclinical study

1. Introduction

Retinitis pigmentosa (RP) is the most common inherited retinal disease, affecting approximately 1 in 4000 individuals worldwide, with an estimated global prevalence of around 3 million people [1]. As its name implies, RP involves the degeneration of retinal cells accompanied by the accumulation of pigments within the retina, leading to its characteristic pigmented appearance. This group of disorders is heterogeneous, encompassing several related conditions such as Leber congenital amaurosis (LCA), Usher syndrome, and Bardet-Biedl syndrome, all of which result in retinal degeneration [1].

RP can be inherited through various modes, including autosomal dominant, autosomal recessive, X-linked recessive, and syndromic inheritance patterns, each associated with distinct mutations, prevalence rates, and disease severity [1–4]. The autosomal recessive form of RP accounts for 50–60% of cases, followed by the autosomal dominant form at 30–40%, and the X-linked form, which constitutes 5–20% of all cases [3, 4]. Despite these genetic variations, the clinical presentation of RP is generally consistent across patients. The disease typically begins with the loss of rod photoreceptors, which are primarily responsible for vision under low-light conditions and are concentrated in the peripheral retina. As these rod cells degenerate, patients initially suffer from night blindness and peripheral vision loss, commonly referred to as "tunnel vision" [3]. Over time, the cone photoreceptors, responsible for central and color vision, are also affected, leading to the gradual loss of central vision. Eventually, most patients with RP become legally blind. These changes are marked by a progressive reduction in the electroretinogram (ERG) response from both rod and cone cells [3].

In addition to vision loss, RP patients often exhibit other ocular abnormalities, including the narrowing of retinal blood vessels, abnormal accumulation of dark, bone-spicule-shaped pigments in the retina, degeneration of the vitreous, and paleness of the optic nerve head [1, 5, 6]. Unfortunately, no definitive and effective treatment for RP currently exists. Available therapies can only slow the progression of retinal degeneration by preserving retinal cell function, reducing cell death, or attempting to replace lost cells through transplantation or artificial means [7]. Pharmacological interventions such as calcium channel blockers, fibroblast growth factor (FGF), and ciliary neurotrophic factor (CTNF) have been explored to modify the retinal environment and prevent further degeneration [8–12]. Additionally, dietary supplements like vitamins A, E, and docosahexaenoic acid (DHA) have been tested as potential treatments [13–15].

In recent years, the success of gene therapy in treating conditions like LCA [NCT00821340, NCT00481546, NCT00749957, NCT02781480, NCT01496040, NCT00643747, NCT04516369, NCT00999609], Choroideremia [NCT03496012], and X-linked RP has raised hopes for the broader application of gene therapy for RP [16–18]. The FDA's 2017 approval of Luxturna (voretigene neparvovec) has further fueled optimism for this therapeutic approach [19, 20].

X-linked RP (XLRP), a particularly severe and rapidly progressing form of RP, has been the focus of recent gene therapy studies. Promising preclinical research has highlighted the potential for gene therapy in treating this condition, although many challenges remain before it can be successfully translated into clinical practice [2, 21–23]. In this review, we aim to explore the genetic basis of XLRP, the preclinical development of gene therapy for this condition, and the current challenges and future directions in the field.

2. X-linked retinitis pigmentosa: A common and severe type of RP

X-linked retinitis pigmentosa (XLRP) is one of the most aggressive forms of RP, known for its early onset and fast progression. Several genetic loci have been associated with XLRP, including RP2 [MIM 312600], RP3 [MIM 312610], RP6 [MIM 312612], RP23 [MIM 300424], RP24 [MIM 300155], and RP34 [MIM 300605]. However, mutations in the RP2 and RPGR (retinitis pigmentosa GTPase regulator) genes are the most studied [3].

RP2 mutations account for approximately 15% of XLRP cases, and they are believed to affect the Golgi apparatus, which is crucial for transporting proteins to the cell surface. Nevertheless, RP2 has been a less frequent target for gene therapy compared to RPGR [24, 25]. Mutations in RPGR, particularly in the ORF15 exon, are responsible for about 70% of XLRP cases and are the most common mutations found in recessive RP. Since the gene is located on the X chromosome, the disease typically affects males, though female carriers may also display varying levels of retinal degeneration, ranging from mild symptoms to severe vision loss resembling the male pattern of the disease [3, 26, 27].

Patients with RPGR mutations often experience early symptoms such as night blindness in childhood, followed by progressive deterioration of both visual acuity and visual fields as photoreceptor cells (rods and cones) die. Most individuals with XLRP are blind by the time they reach their forties. Optical coherence tomography (OCT) imaging shows that these patients tend to have progressive thinning of the outer retinal layers [28, 29].

3. Genetic pathology

The RPGR gene, located on Xp21.1, spans approximately 58 kb and comprises 19 exons. During transcription, 10 different mRNA isoforms are produced through alternative splicing, with five of these being translated into proteins. The two most prominent forms of RPGR mRNA are RPGREx1-19, which encodes a 2448 bp protein with 815 amino acids, and RPGRORF15, which includes the first 14 exons followed by an extension of the 15th exon and a 3459 bp sequence encoding a protein of 1152 amino acids [1].

RPGR is expressed in two primary isoforms: RPGRconst, which is present in various tissues throughout the body, and RPGRORF15, which is specifically expressed in photoreceptor cells [30]. The exact function of RPGR is not fully understood, but it is believed to play a role in the transport of proteins between the inner and outer segments of photoreceptor cells. These segments are essential for the normal functioning of the retina, as they are involved in the retinoid cycle that underpins vision [31, 32].

Mutations in the final exon, ORF15, represent a mutational hotspot, accounting for over 70% of RPGR mutations. The repetitive sequences in this region are prone to forming abnormal DNA conformations that disrupt the transcription and translation of the RPGR gene [30, 33]. Most mutations in ORF15 are small deletions of 1–5 base pairs, which cause a frameshift and lead to the truncation of the RPGR protein.

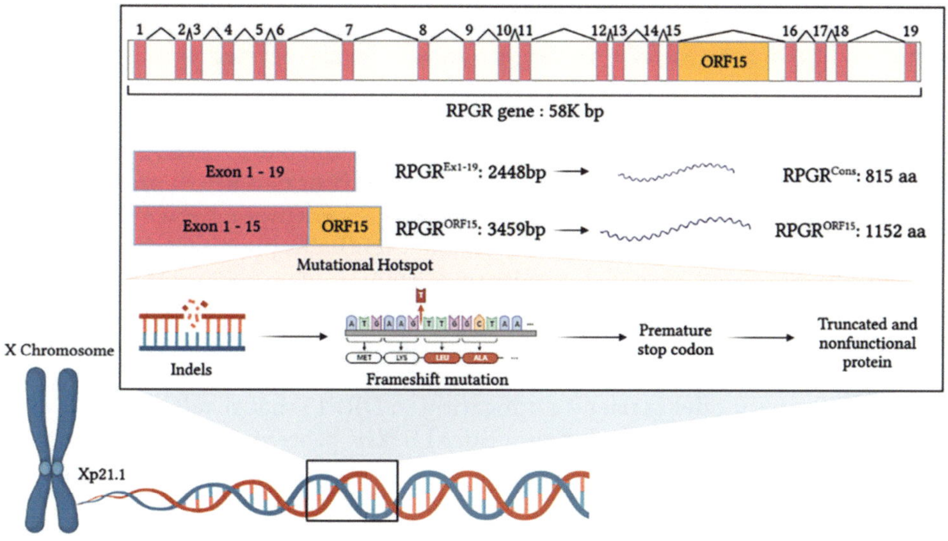

Figure 1.
Schematic diagram of retinitis pigmentosa GTPase regulator (RPGR) gene structure, splicing variants, and genetic pathogenesis of XLRP.

This can disrupt protein stability and function, eventually leading to photoreceptor degeneration due to altered isoelectric balance and impaired post-translational modifications [30, 34–36].

Interestingly, small non-frameshift deletions in ORF15 can be tolerated and may even improve genome stability. It is also notable that the RPGREx1-19 isoform does not compensate for the loss of RPGRORF15 function in the retina, as it is only minimally expressed in this tissue [37–39]. **Figure 1** provides a visual representation of this process.

4. Animal models of XLRP disease

One of the essential components for testing the safety and efficacy of RPGR gene therapy is the availability of suitable animal models that can accurately replicate the features and progression of XLRP seen in humans. These models play a critical role in preclinical research, aiding in the selection of viral vectors and gene therapy designs. Retinal degenerative diseases affect various species, and many of the genes that cause retinal degeneration in animals are homologous to those implicated in human retinal diseases. This allows for the development of animal models that are both genetically and phenotypically analogous to human conditions [1].

Animal models for XLRP fall into two categories: those with naturally occurring RPGR mutations and those that have been genetically engineered. A wide range of animals, including dogs, mice, rats, cats, chickens, and pigs, have been used to model retinal diseases. Dogs and pigs, in particular, are valuable models due to their retinal size and anatomical similarities to humans. Cats are also favored due to their well-documented retinal neurophysiology and lower inflammation rates following ocular interventions [1].

The most common XLRP models, however, are murine. Mice are advantageous because they have a relatively short lifespan, allowing researchers to observe disease progression in a shorter time frame. Although mice have smaller eyes, which complicates certain procedures, they breed quickly, making them ideal for large-scale genetic studies. In contrast, rats are larger and have better-defined photoreceptors, but their longer lifespan can slow down research [1].

Three animal models with natural RPGR mutations are widely studied: the XLPRA1 and XLPRA2 canine models and the rd9 mouse model. XLPRA1 is caused by a five-nucleotide deletion in ORF15, resulting in a truncated RPGR protein, which leads to progressive degeneration of the retina. Rod degeneration begins around 11 months of age, followed by cone cell loss, and eventually, photoreceptor function is lost [40]. In the XLPRA2 model, a more severe mutation results in a frameshift mutation that creates a truncated protein with altered amino acid composition. This model exhibits rapid retinal degeneration, with photoreceptor loss beginning around 4 weeks of age [40].

The rd9 mouse model carries a duplication in ORF15 that results in a frameshift mutation, leading to a loss of functional RPGR protein. Retinal degeneration in rd9 mice is gradual, with the outer nuclear layer thinning and reduced rhodopsin and transducin levels in the rod cells. ERG responses gradually decline, and pigmentary changes appear with age [41, 42]. Additionally, several genetically engineered models have been developed to study XLRP, including RPGR-knockout mice, which have early-onset retinal degeneration similar to that observed in XLRP patients [43].

While the canine models are particularly useful due to their large eyes, making them amenable to surgical interventions similar to those used in humans, murine models remain indispensable for understanding the molecular mechanisms of XLRP and for large-scale screening studies. The choice of model depends on the specific research goals, whether they are focused on therapeutic development or disease mechanism studies.

5. Gene therapy vectors

The successful application of gene therapy depends not only on selecting appropriate animal models but also on choosing the optimal viral vector for delivering the therapeutic gene. **Figure 2** shows different elements of retinal gene therapy strategies.

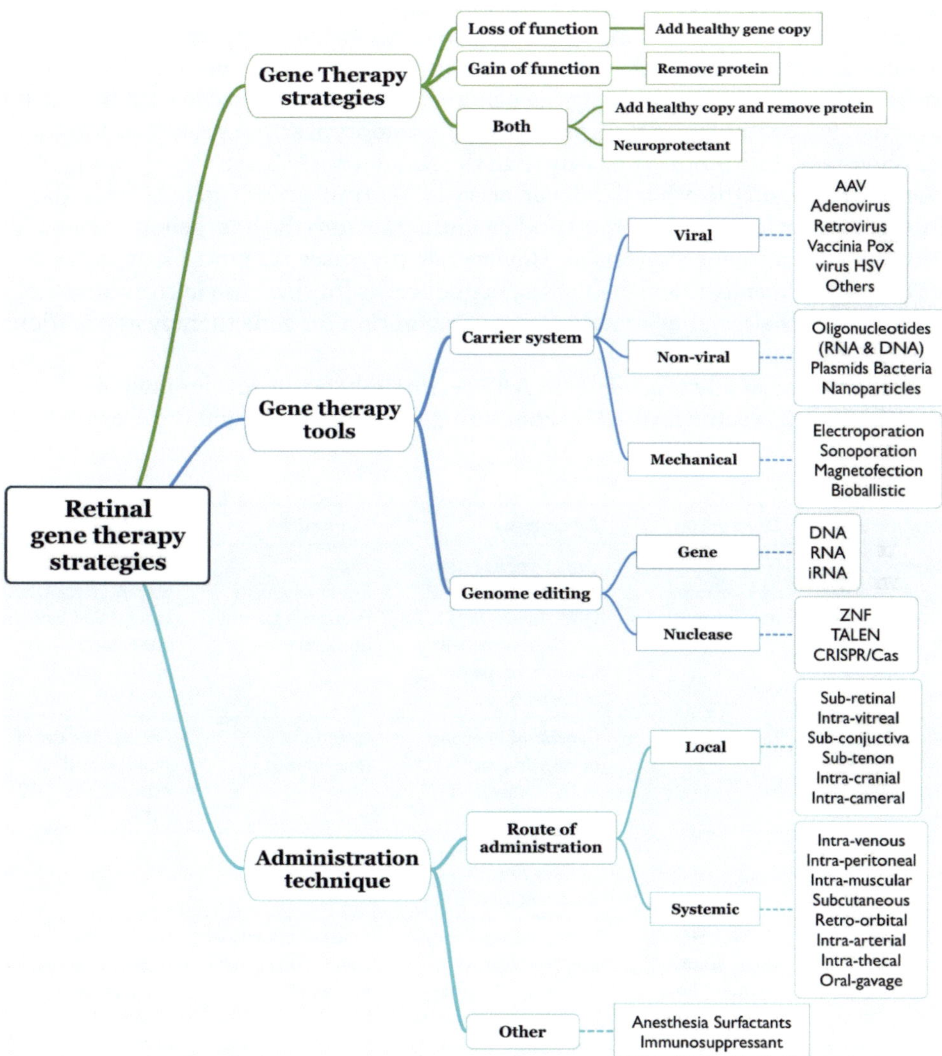

Figure 2.
Retinal gene therapy strategies and their components. Each component is crucial in designing retinal gene therapies.

In each gene therapy, an appropriate vector type should be selected according to these elements. Viral vectors have been the most commonly used gene transfer tools in gene therapy trials due to their high efficiency and ability to transduce a variety of cells. Among the different viral vectors, adeno-associated viruses (AAVs) and lentiviruses are the most frequently used for ocular gene therapy [44]. **Table 1** summarizes the advantages and disadvantages of these vectors.

AAVs have become particularly popular in ocular gene therapy because they are non-pathogenic and elicit minimal immune responses. Moreover, AAVs can transduce both dividing and non-dividing cells, which is advantageous for retinal cells. These vectors can either integrate into the host genome at a known locus, reducing the risk of insertional mutagenesis, or remain episomal, enabling long-term transgene expression without altering the host DNA [45, 46].

Different AAV serotypes show varying tropisms for ocular cells. AAV2, AAV5, and AAV8 are most effective at targeting photoreceptor cells, while AAV1 and AAV2 are more efficient at transducing retinal pigment epithelial (RPE) cells [47, 48]. To enhance the transduction efficiency and specificity of AAVs, pseudotyped vectors have been developed by combining the genome of one AAV serotype with the capsid of another. For example, AAV2/5 and AAV2/8 pseudotypes have been found to transduce photoreceptors more efficiently than the standard AAV2 serotype [49–51].

Lentiviruses, on the other hand, can carry larger transgenes (up to 11 kb in the third-generation lentiviral vectors) and can integrate into the host genome, ensuring long-term transgene expression. However, lentiviruses are more likely to cause insertional mutagenesis, which raises safety concerns for their use in clinical settings [44, 52]. Nevertheless, they remain a promising option for gene therapy applications that require larger gene payloads.

One of the latest advancements in AAV technology is the development of AAV-DJ, a hybrid vector formed by combining the capsids of eight different AAV

Viral vector	Description	Advantages	Limitations	Applications
Adenoviruses	Non-enveloped, 36 kb genome, non-integrative	Capable of insertion of large fragments of DNA, infection of a large variety of cells, and easy propagation in the body	High immunogenicity (both cellular and humoral)	Transient expression of transgenes, DNA vaccine development due to high immunogenicity
Retroviruses (including lentiviruses)	Integrative	Capable of insertion of large fragments of DNA, low immunogenicity, infection of both proliferating and quiescent cells	Insertional mutagenesis	Genetic diseases of T cells including malignancies, HIV/AIDS
Adeno-associated virus (AAV)	Non-enveloped, single-stranded DNA, 4.7 kb genome, either integrative or non-integrative	low immunogenicity, easy propagation in the body, infection of a large variety of cells, long-term gene expression	Limited capacity for transferring genetic materials	Genetic diseases, tumors, neurological, ocular, and cardiovascular diseases

Table 1.
Advantages and disadvantages of the leading viral vectors used for gene therapy of eye diseases.

serotypes. This vector has demonstrated enhanced transduction efficiency across a broader range of cell types, making it a valuable tool for both *in vitro* and *in vivo* applications [53, 54].

In clinical trials for inherited retinal diseases, AAV has been the most widely used vector, with AAV2 and AAV8 being particularly favored. Only in a few cases have lentiviral vectors been used, mainly due to AAV's limited packaging capacity, which is insufficient for larger genes. Antisense oligonucleotides have also been explored to modulate gene expression at the mRNA level in some trials [55, 56]. Given the relative safety and efficiency of AAV vectors, they remain the primary choice for ongoing and future ocular gene therapy research [44, 57].

6. Preclinical gene therapy trials of XLRP

Over the past decade, several preclinical studies have explored gene therapy as a potential treatment for X-linked retinitis pigmentosa (XLRP), with promising results. These studies primarily focus on delivering a functional copy of the RPGR gene using adeno-associated virus (AAV) vectors. One of the first notable studies, conducted in 2012, involved the use of an AAV5 vector to deliver the RPGR gene under the control of either the interphotoreceptor retinoid-binding protein (IRBP) promoter or the human G-protein-coupled receptor kinase 1 (hGRK1) promoter. This therapy was administered subretinally in two canine models of XLRP and successfully preserved rod and cone photoreceptor function [58].

In 2015, another study investigated RPGR gene replacement in RPGR-knockout mice (RPGR−/−) using an AAV vector. The gene was delivered under the control of a rhodopsin kinase promoter, and the treated mice showed improved electroretinogram (ERG) responses and preservation of retinal layers. This study also explored the effects of different vector doses, highlighting the need to carefully balance viral load to avoid potential side effects associated with higher doses [59].

Another preclinical study, conducted on a canine model carrying a natural RPGR mutation (XLPRA2), evaluated the therapeutic effects of different doses of AAV2 and AAV5 vectors expressing RPGR. The study examined the expression of RPGR protein, immune responses, and structural changes in the retina, such as photoreceptor thickness and opsin localization. The results demonstrated superior performance with the rAAV2tYF-GRK1-hRPGRco vector, offering insights into dose optimization for future human trials [60].

Recent advances in CRISPR/Cas9 technology have also been explored for XLRP gene therapy. Preclinical studies using the RPGR −/y mouse model employed CRISPR/Cas9 to repair the RPGR gene *via* homology-directed repair (HDR). These studies demonstrated therapeutic benefits lasting 6–12 months post-treatment, further supporting the potential of gene editing techniques for treating retinal degenerative diseases [61, 62].

A summary of these preclinical gene therapy trials can be found in **Table 2**. The most commonly used animal models in these studies are rd9 mice and the XLPRA2 canine model. AAV2/5 and AAV2/8 are the preferred vectors, and CRISPR/Cas9 technology has shown promise in both gene repair and disease reversal. However, challenges remain in achieving stable RPGR expression and uniform vector distribution across the retina following subretinal injection. The retinal toxicity observed with high vector doses further emphasizes the need for careful dose-finding studies during preclinical assessments. Future research should also explore vectors with engineered

Authors	Year	Animal model	Agent and gene	Dosage	Findings
Hong et al. [63]	2005	RPGR-knockout (KO) mice	Shortened RPGR cDNA	Transfected into mouse embryonic stem cells. Transgenic chimeras were crossed with RPGR-KO mice	• Expression of RPGR-ORF15 in rods and cones • Rescue of function and structure of retinal degeneration
Beltran et al. [58]	2012	XLPRA1 and XLPRA2 canine models	AAV 2/5–vectored human RPGR with human IRBP or GRK1 promoters	1.05×10^{10} vg in 70 μL at 5th week, 21.25×10^{10} vg in 150 μL at 28th week	• preserved photoreceptor nuclei and inner/outer segments • improved rod and cone photoreceptor function • reversal of opsin mislocalization
Wu et al. [59]	2015	Rpgr-KO mice	AAV8-mRpgr (mouse RPGR), AAV8-hRPGR (human RPGR) and AAV9-mRpgr (mouse RPGR)	1×10^{11} to 1×10^{13} in 1 μL	• maintained the expression of RPGR-ORF15 throughout the study duration • Better electroretinogram response • remarkable preservation of retinal structure and function • Retinal toxicity was observed at high vector doses needing dose optimization
Beltran et al. [64, 65]	2015	XLPRA2 dogs	AAV2/5 vector construct carrying full-length human RPGR1-ORF15 cDNA under control of a hIRBP promoter	70–150 μL at the concentration of 1.51×10^{11} vg/ml	• Earlier intervention results in better results • Preserved therapeutic function of intervention • Significant improvement in structural, functional and behavioral assessments
Mookherjee et al. [66]	2015	Rp2-KO mice	AAV8-scRK-hRP2	1×10^{8}, 3×10^{8} or 1×10^{9} vector genomes	• Preservation of cone function, viability • Correction of opsin trafficking • Retinal toxicity in high-dose group
Deng et al. [67]	2015	C57/B mice	AAV-hIRBP-hRPGR and AAV-hGRK1-hRPGR	1μl of AAV at low dose of 10^{10} vg/ml, mid dose of 1.5×10^{11} vg/ml and high dose of 10^{13} vg/ml	• Expression of RPGR • No retinal toxicity
Pawlyk et al. [39]	2016	Rpgr−/− mice	AAV2/8-RK-ORF15-L and AAV2/8-RK-ORF15-S	2×10^{9} vg or 5×10^{9} vg	• Significant functional and morphological rescue of rods and cones in long RPGR form • More stability in shorter form while remaining functional

Authors	Year	Animal model	Agent and gene	Dosage	Findings
Fischer et al. [22]	2017	Two Mouse models (Rpgr−/y and C57BL/6JRd9/Boc)	AAV 2/8 encoding for RPGRORF15 with photoreceptor-specific human rhodopsin kinase (RK) promoter	1.5×10^9 vg in 1.5 μL	• Optimized gene replacement therapy with stable production of the full-length RPGR protein • Preserved glutamulation properties of RPGR following codon optimization • Acceptable safety in animals • Rescued function of rod and cone receptors
Beltran et al. [21]	2017	XLPRA2 canine models, macaques (Macaca mulatta and Macaca fascicularis)	AAV2/5 vector carrying hRPGRstb and hRPGRco under control of GRK1 and IRBP promoters	70–100 μL at the concentration of 1.5×10^{11} and 1.5×10^{12} vg/mL	• Ability of AAV 2/5 to transduct both rod and cone receptors • Efficiency of GRK1 and IRBP promoters for rescuing photoreceptors
Giacalone et al. [68]	2019	wild-type Sprague Dawley rats	AAV 2/5-CMV-IA-RPGR	10 μL of at the concentration of 1×10^{12} vg/mL	• Stable expression of mutant RPGR • Functional RPGR transcript and protein production
Schlegel et al. [69]	2019	B6J.Sv129-Rpgrtm1Sti	AAV2/5.CMV.I-SceI-T2A-GFP and AAV2/8.RK.I-SceI-T2A-GFP	1 μL each of vector at the concentration of 3×10^{11} vg/mL	• Proof of concept of a human-XLRP gene therapy using endonuclease I-SceI
Song et al. [60]	2020	XLPRA2 canine model	rAAV2tYF-GRK1-hRPGRco or rAAV2tYF-GRK1-hRPGRstb	150 μL at the concentration of 3.0×10^{12} vg/mL (High Dose), 6.0×10^{11} vg/mL (Mid Dose), or 1.2×10^{11} vg/mL (Low Dose)	• No significant signs of ocular discomfort or ophthalmic complications • Rescue the function and structure of photoreceptors • Stronger expression for rAAV2tYF-GRK1-hRP-GRco compared to rAAV2tYF-GRK1-hRPGRstb • Correction of rod and cone opsin mislocalization
Hu et al. [62]	2020	Rpgr−/yCas9+/WT mice	AAV 2/8 encoding for sgRNA targeted to the mutant Rpgr locus and donor template	1 μL at a concentration of 1×10^{12} vector genomes per milliliter	• Significant photoreceptor preservation • Therapeutic effect lasts for up to 12 months with no off-target effects

Authors	Year	Animal model	Agent and gene	Dosage	Findings
Dufour et al. [70]	2020	XLPRA2 dog model	AAV2tYF with GRK1 promoter	0.07 mL at the concentration of low (1.2×10^{11} vg/mL), mid (6×10^{11} vg/mL), or high dose (3×10^{12} vg/mL)	• Well toleration without systemic toxicity • Rescue of functional and structural of photoreceptors • Posterior segment toxicity at high dose level
Gumerson et al. [61]	2022	Rd9 mice	Dual AAV vectors: one containing SpCas9 driven by RK promoter and another containing both the RPGR-targeted sgRNA driven by the U6 promoter and tdTomato reporter gene driven by RK promoter	1 μl of each vector at the concentration of 7.5×10^9–1×10^{10} vg/μl	• Restored reading frame of RPGRORF15 • Broad distribution throughout the retina following subretinal injection

Table 2.
The characteristics and findings of preclinical trials of X-linked Retinitis pigmentosa gene therapy.

capsids that can penetrate retinal layers after intravitreal injection, providing a less invasive approach to gene delivery.

7. Gene therapy clinical trials of XLRP

In recent years, several clinical trials have been initiated to assess the safety and efficacy of gene therapy for XLRP. While the number of trials is growing, results from many of these studies are still pending. A notable first-in-human phase 1/2 clinical trial using an AAV8 vector encoding a codon-optimized human RPGR gene demonstrated promising results, showing both safety and sustained improvements in visual fields [2].

Another phase 1/2 study employed an AAV5 vector expressing RPGRORF15 under the control of the human rhodopsin kinase (hRK) promoter. This study reported clinically meaningful improvements in photoreceptor function and sensitivity at 12 months post-injection [71].

As outlined in **Table 3**, gene therapy for XLRP is now entering phase 3 trials. Given the progress made so far, the approval of a gene therapy product for XLRP in the near future seems increasingly likely. Early clinical trial results provide hope that gene therapy can not only halt the progression of retinal degeneration but also restore some degree of visual function in affected patients.

7.1 Evaluations and measurements

Accurate and comprehensive evaluation methods are essential for assessing the baseline characteristics of retinal degeneration and monitoring the outcomes of gene therapy interventions. These assessments should capture both functional and structural changes in the retina, which are crucial for determining the efficacy of the treatment. Functional evaluations typically include optomotor (optokinetic) testing, electrophysiology, and visual evoked potentials (VEP), while structural assessments are done using methods such as ophthalmoscopy, optical coherence tomography (OCT), histology, and immunofluorescence [17].

Functional and structural evaluations are complementary, providing a full picture of how the retina responds to gene therapy. For example, OCT can reveal the morphological changes in retinal layers, while ERG and VEP provide information about the functionality of photoreceptors and the visual system as a whole. The combination of these approaches enables researchers and clinicians to detect subtle changes and track disease progression, as well as the effects of therapy on both rod and cone cells [21, 22].

7.2 Functional assessments

7.2.1 Optomotor test

The optomotor test measures an animal's spatial visual function based on its optokinetic response. The test involves presenting the animal with a rotating visual stimulus, such as alternating dark and light stripes on the inner surface of a cylinder. As the stripes move, the animal instinctively follows the stimulus with head movements. The experimenter observes whether the animal's head movements are synchronized with the rotating pattern, indicating that the animal can detect the stimulus [72].

NCT number	Intervention/Observation	Design	Number of participants	Start/Finish year	Clinical center(s)	Sponsor
NCT03116113	Subretinal delivery of AAV8-hRKcoRPGRORF15 (BIIB112)	A multicenter, open-label dose Escalation (Phase 1), and Dose Expansion (Phase 2/3) Clinical Trial (XIRIUS Trial)	Phase 1: 18 participants/Phase 2: 63 participants	March 2017/ November 2020	Oxford, Manchester, Southampton, UK, Florida, Oregon, Pennsylvania, USA	Nightstar Therapeutics (now Biogen Inc), UK
NCT03252847	Subretinal delivery of AAV2/5-hRKRPGRORF15	An Open-Label, Multi-center, Phase I/II Dose Escalation Trial	36 participants	July 2017/ November 2021 (no reports yet)	London, UK	MeiraGTx, UK
NCT03316560	Subretinal delivery of rAAV2tYFGRK1-coRPGRORF15	a non-randomized, open-label, Phase 1/2 dose escalation study, with a phase 2 randomized, controlled, masked dose expansion study	Phase 1/2: 30 participants/Phase 2: 12 participants	April 2018/ August 2026	Colorado, Massachusetts, New York, North Carolina, Ohio, Oregon, Pennsylvania, Texas, USA	Applied Genetic Technologies Corporation (AGTC), USA
NCT04850118	rAAV2tYF-GRK1-hRPGRco (AGTC-501)	A Phase 2/3, Randomized, Controlled, Masked, Multicenter Study	63 participants	August 2021/ March 2029	Applied Genetic Technologies Corp	Applied Genetic Technologies Corp
NCT04671433	AAV5-RPGR	Phase 3 Randomized, Controlled Study	66 participants	March 2021/July 2022	California, Florida, Georgia, Massachusetts, Michigan, Texas, USA	MeiraGTx UK II Ltd., Janssen Research & Development, LLC
NCT04517149	4D-125	An Open-label, Phase 1/2 Trial	43 participants	June 2020/May 2029	Colorado, Florida, Michigan, North Carolina, Oregon, Texas, Utah, USA	4D Molecular Therapeutics
NCT04794101	AAV5-RPGR	Follow-up phase 3 Randomized, Controlled Study	66 participants	March 2021/July 2027	California, Florida, Georgia, Massachusetts, Michigan, Texas, USA	MeiraGTx UK II Ltd., Janssen Research & Development, LLC
NCT04312672	AAV2-RPGR	Follow-Up Study of an Open-Label, Multi-Center, Phase I/II Dose Escalation Trial	36 participants	February 2019/ June 2023	London, UK	MeiraGTx UK II Ltd
NCT03584165	Subretinal delivery of AAV8-hRKcoRPGRORF15 (BIIB112)	A Long-term Follow-up phase 3 Study	440 participants	June 2018/ March 2027	Multiple centers in the UK, Netherlands, Germany, France, Finland, Denmark, Canada, USA	NightstaRx Ltd., a Biogen Company

NCT number	Intervention/Observation	Design	Number of participants	Start/Finish year	Clinical center(s)	Sponsor
NCT03349242	Prospective natural history study of XLRP	Observational study	250 participants	December 2017/ December 2023	Massachusetts, Michigan, USA	MeiraGTx, UK
NCT03314207	Prospective natural history study of XLRP caused by RPGR-ORF15 mutations	Observational study	45 participants	December 2017/ December 2021	New York, North Carolina, Ohio, Oregon, Texas, USA	Applied Genetic Technologies Corporation (AGTC), USA

Table 3.
Summary of clinical trials for RPGR-related X-linked retinitis pigmentosa (XLRP).

In the second part of the test, various sinusoidal patterns with different frequencies and contrasts are shown to determine the animal's visual thresholds (**Figure 3**) [73].

This test assesses both the visual and motor systems. For example, in mouse models of RP, optomotor thresholds decrease as the disease progresses, reflecting photoreceptor degeneration. Rescue of photoreceptor function through gene therapy has been shown to restore these thresholds [66].

7.2.2 Electrophysiological assessments

The electroretinogram (ERG) is one of the most widely used tools to assess photoreceptor function. ERG measures the electrical response of retinal cells to light stimuli, allowing researchers to evaluate the function of rods and cones separately. The results are presented as two waveforms: the "a" wave, representing the initial response of photoreceptors, and the "b" wave, which corresponds to the activity of bipolar cells in the retina [74].

RP is typically classified as a rod-cone disorder, with rod cells being affected earlier in the disease course. Over time, the amplitude of the ERG waveforms declines as the retinal area becomes progressively dysfunctional [75]. The ERG is particularly useful for diagnosing RP and assessing the overall health of the retina, though its ability to detect subtle changes in localized regions, such as the macula, is limited [76]. In XLRP animal models, ERG wave amplitudes decrease with age, but gene therapy has been shown to halt the decline and improve the timing and intensity of ERG waveforms [41, 77–79].

7.2.3 Visual evoked potentials (VEP)

VEPs measure the electrical responses of the visual cortex to visual stimuli. Electrodes are placed on the scalp to record the brain's response to a visual stimulus, providing insight into the function of the entire visual pathway, from the retina to

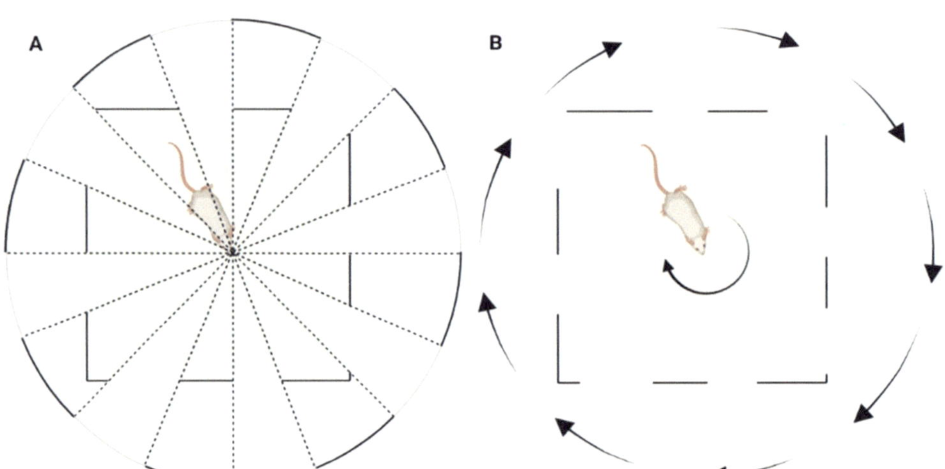

Figure 3.
Schema of the optomotor test. (A) A virtual rotating cylinder consisting of black and white grid lines around the animal is shown in part A. (B) Animal head movement should be consistent with the rotation of the virtual cylinder.

the brain. In RP patients, VEP measurements show delayed response times (increased latency) and reduced amplitudes, reflecting the loss of photoreceptor function and the disruption of visual signal transmission [80–83].

While VEP is not as widely used in preclinical studies of RP as ERG, it can be a valuable tool for assessing changes in visual signal transmission, particularly when combined with ERG recordings, to pinpoint which part of the visual system is most affected [84].

7.3 Structural and morphological assessments

7.3.1 Optical coherence tomography (OCT)

Optical coherence tomography (OCT) is a non-invasive imaging technique that allows for detailed visualization of retinal layers. OCT has become a vital tool for both clinical and preclinical studies of retinal diseases, enabling the detection of subtle structural changes in the retina. The development of spectral domain OCT (SD-OCT) has significantly improved the resolution of these images, providing a micrometer-scale view of retinal layers, which can closely correlate with histological findings [17, 85].

In patients with retinitis pigmentosa (RP), OCT imaging reveals various changes, such as thinning of the outer nuclear layer (ONL), disruptions in the external limiting membrane (ELM) and ellipsoid zone (EZ), and the development of cystoid macular edema or epiretinal membranes [86–91]. These observations are also used to monitor the progression of the disease and response to treatments like gene therapy. In preclinical studies, OCT can be used with animal models to track retinal degeneration and therapeutic outcomes. For example, murine models of RP show thinning of the ONL and disorganization of photoreceptor layers on OCT imaging as the disease progresses [92]. Gene therapy targeting RPGR in XLRP models has been shown to preserve ONL thickness and improve the structural integrity of the retina (**Figure 4**) [21, 22, 42].

7.3.2 Histology

Histological analysis provides a deeper understanding of the cellular and tissue-level changes that occur during retinal degeneration. This method involves examining retinal sections under a microscope to assess the structure of photoreceptor cells and the overall organization of retinal layers. Immunofluorescence and immunocytochemistry are also commonly used to label specific proteins and visualize their distribution within the retina [41, 93].

For example, immunofluorescence staining for RPGR protein in XLRP animal models reveals mislocalization of the protein in the photoreceptor connecting cilia, a key feature of the disease [34]. After gene therapy, the RPGR protein is restored to its correct location, accumulating between the inner and outer segments of the photoreceptors, which closely resembles the arrangement in healthy cells [39]. Histological analysis also allows researchers to count the number of photoreceptor cells and measure ONL thickness, providing a quantitative assessment of retinal degeneration and recovery following treatment.

7.3.3 Ophthalmoscopy of the lens and fundus (with ophthalmoscope or slit lamp)

Ophthalmoscopy is used to examine the retina for visible signs of disease, such as pigmentary changes, retinal vessel narrowing, and other abnormalities that indicate retinal degeneration. In animal models of RP, fundus imaging reveals characteristic

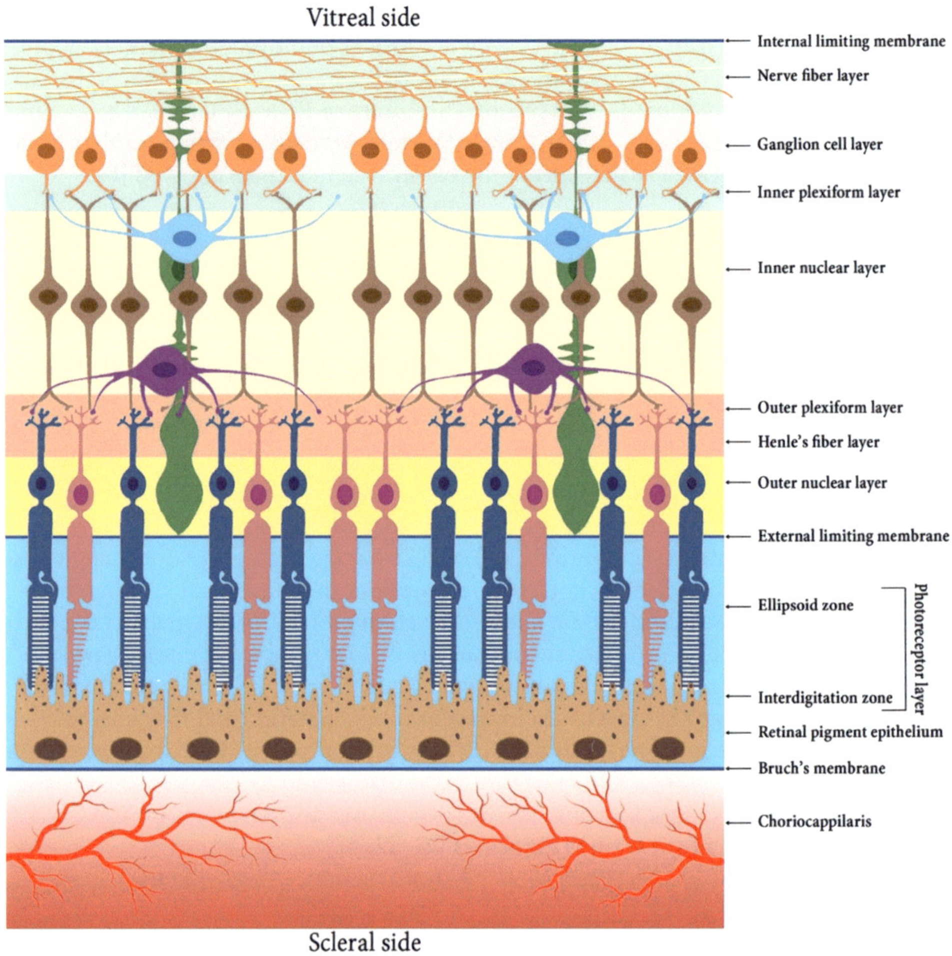

Figure 4.
The schematic illustration of retinal cell layers.

bone-spicule pigmentation and attenuated retinal vessels, which are hallmarks of the disease [94]. Slit lamp examination may also detect the presence of posterior subcapsular cataracts, which are commonly observed in RP patients [95]. In heterozygous female carriers of XLRP, ophthalmoscopy may reveal patchy retinal degeneration, reflecting random X-inactivation and variable expression of the mutant allele [96].

7.3.4 Retinal angiography

Fluorescein-assisted retinal angiography is occasionally used to evaluate retinal blood vessels. Although this technique is used less frequently in modern practice, it can still provide valuable information about retinal vascular attenuation, a common feature of RP [94].

7.3.5 Immunoblotting

Immunoblotting is a method used to detect specific proteins in the retina, such as RPGR, by separating them based on size and charge and then using antibodies for identification. This technique is particularly useful for studying protein expression in animal models of XLRP and assessing the effects of gene therapy on RPGR expression levels [31, 34].

8. Challenges in RPGR gene therapy

Despite the promising advances in gene therapy for XLRP, several significant challenges remain that must be addressed to improve therapeutic outcomes.

8.1 Manufacturing instability of ORF15

The ORF15 region of the RPGR gene is a mutational hotspot, and its instability during recombination and manufacturing processes has posed a major hurdle for gene therapy development. ORF15 is a purine-rich region, which makes it prone to forming abnormal DNA structures, leading to transcription and translation errors [30]. Approximately 80% of mutations in the RPGR gene are located in ORF15, and these mutations are often small deletions that cause frameshift mutations, resulting in truncated proteins [97]. Additionally, it has been observed that the complete deletion of ORF15 interferes with RPGR function, but moderate shortening of this sequence may increase stability without compromising protein function [39].

To address these challenges, researchers have optimized the RPGRORF15 coding sequence (CDS) for gene therapy. This optimization includes reducing the frequency of codons for rare amino acids, removing problematic sequences such as poly-T and poly-A repeats, and enhancing GC content to increase mRNA stability. These modifications help prevent issues during the recombination process and improve the stability of the gene therapy product [2, 22].

8.2 Route of vector injection

Another significant challenge in RPGR gene therapy is determining the optimal route for delivering viral vectors to the retina. Two common methods are subretinal injection and intravitreal injection, each with its own advantages and drawbacks.

In the subretinal injection approach, the vector is delivered directly into the space between the retina and the RPE, providing efficient access to the photoreceptors. However, this method can induce retinal detachment and inflammation, although these effects are usually temporary and manageable with corticosteroids [2, 98, 99]. Subretinal injections are more invasive and pose a higher risk of surgical complications, which emphasizes the importance of surgeon expertise [100].

Intravitreal injection, on the other hand, is less invasive and associated with fewer complications. However, due to the longer distance between the injection site and the target photoreceptor cells, the efficacy of this approach is limited [98]. In recent years, engineered AAV capsids, such as AAV pseudotypes and AAV-DJ, have been developed to improve vector penetration through retinal layers after intravitreal injection, offering a less invasive alternative for gene therapy delivery [48, 101].

8.3 Distribution of vectors across the retina

One of the challenges with subretinal injections is the limited distribution of viral vectors, which tends to be confined to the area of the retina around the injection site. This restricted distribution can result in uneven treatment effects. Researchers are exploring new delivery methods, such as viral vector scaffolds, to achieve more uniform distribution across the retina [98, 102]. Intravitreal injection, while offering more widespread distribution within the inner retina, faces the obstacle of the inner limiting membrane, which prevents viral vectors from reaching the outer photoreceptor layers in larger animals and humans [44].

8.4 Timing of gene therapy

Another challenge is identifying the optimal time for administering gene therapy. Studies have shown that the efficacy of gene therapy varies depending on the stage of disease progression. Administering therapy early in the disease course, before significant photoreceptor loss has occurred, appears to be more effective [103]. This highlights the importance of early diagnosis and timely intervention to maximize the benefits of gene therapy.

8.5 Optimizing transgenes

Finally, the complexity of the RPGR gene, particularly the ORF15 region, presents a challenge for gene therapy. The AG-rich sequences in ORF15 can disrupt mRNA splicing and create instability during recombination. To address this, several studies have optimized the RPGRORF15 sequence by removing splicing signals, reducing codon repetition, and stabilizing the mRNA structure. These changes have improved the efficiency and stability of the therapeutic transgene [2, 22].

9. The future of RPGR gene therapy

Although Luxturna (voretigene neparvovec) is the only gene therapy approved for retinal diseases as of now, the rapidly growing field of RPGR gene therapy holds considerable promise for the treatment of X-linked retinitis pigmentosa (XLRP). The progress made in preclinical studies and early-phase clinical trials has generated optimism about the potential for gene therapy to halt or even reverse the progression of XLRP in the near future.

However, several challenges remain. The first is the optimization of the RPGR gene sequence, particularly the unstable ORF15 region, which is prone to mutations and errors during recombination processes [97]. Advances in gene synthesis and vector engineering are gradually overcoming these barriers. For instance, shortening and optimizing the ORF15 sequence has been shown to maintain protein function while improving stability during manufacturing [37].

Another area of focus is the development of viral vectors with better distribution and transduction efficiency. Current AAV vectors have shown great promise in targeting photoreceptor cells, but improvements in the capsid structure of AAV vectors—such as hybrid vectors like AAV-DJ—could further enhance the delivery of therapeutic genes to the retina, particularly when using less invasive delivery routes like intravitreal injection [53, 54]. Additionally, future research should focus on improving the uniformity of vector distribution across the retina to ensure consistent therapeutic effects [98].

As research continues to move forward, several clinical trials for XLRP gene therapy have reached advanced phases, making the approval of a gene therapy product for this condition highly plausible in the near future. However, long-term studies are essential to evaluate the durability of gene therapy outcomes and to monitor potential side effects, such as immune responses to the viral vectors used.

With the ongoing refinement of gene therapy techniques, there is potential not only for treating XLRP but also for addressing a wide range of inherited retinal diseases. The future of RPGR gene therapy looks promising, and further developments in vector design, delivery methods, and gene editing technologies like CRISPR/Cas9 are likely to play a significant role in shaping the future of retinal gene therapies [61].

10. Conclusions

In summary, gene therapy for X-linked retinitis pigmentosa (XLRP) has made substantial progress in recent years, driven by advancements in viral vector development, animal models, and genetic engineering technologies. Mutations in the RPGR gene, particularly in the ORF15 region, are the primary cause of XLRP, and gene therapy targeting this gene has shown great promise in preclinical models and early-stage clinical trials [30, 39]. However, challenges such as vector distribution, gene stability, and the timing of intervention remain.

Current research is focused on addressing these obstacles through the optimization of gene sequences, the development of more efficient viral vectors, and the refinement of delivery methods. Early intervention and personalized approaches based on genetic testing could significantly enhance the efficacy of these treatments.

The future of RPGR gene therapy holds great promise, with the potential to provide a long-lasting solution for patients suffering from XLRP. As ongoing clinical trials progress, we may soon see a gene therapy product specifically designed for XLRP entering the market, offering hope to individuals facing vision loss from this devastating disease.

Conflict of interest

The authors declare no "conflict of interest."

Declarations

This chapter incorporates content and findings from our previously published manuscript titled "X-Linked Retinitis Pigmentosa Gene Therapy: Preclinical Aspects" [104]. This manuscript is licensed under a Creative Commons Attribution-NonCommercial 4.0 International License, which permits non-commercial use, sharing, adaptation, distribution, and reproduction in any medium or format, provided that appropriate credit is given to the original authors and source, a link to the Creative Commons license is provided. Some minor changes have been made to meet the IntechOpen template guideline for chapters. Any images or third-party materials included in the previous manuscript are covered under the same license unless otherwise stated. For further details on the licensing agreement, please refer to [105] the link: [Creative Commons License] (http://creativecommons.org/licenses/by-nc/4.0/).

Author details

Vahid Mansouri* and Maryam Bemanalizadeh
Gene Therapy Research Center, Shariati Hospital, Tehran University of Medical Sciences, Tehran, Iran

*Address all correspondence to: mansoury.vahid@gmail.com

References

[1] Rivas MA, Vecino E. Animal models and different therapies for treatment of retinitis pigmentosa. Histology and Histopathology. 2009;**24**(10):1295-1322

[2] Cehajic-Kapetanovic J, Xue K, Martinez-Fernandez de la Camara C, Nanda A, Davies A, Wood LJ, et al. Initial results from a first-in-human gene therapy trial on X-linked retinitis pigmentosa caused by mutations in RPGR. Nature Medicine. 2020;**26**(3):354-359

[3] Petrs-Silva H, Linden R. Advances in gene therapy technologies to treat retinitis pigmentosa. Clinical Ophthalmology. 2014;**8**:127-136. DOI: 10.2147/OPTH.S38041

[4] Sahel J, Bonnel S, Mrejen S, Paques M. Retinitis pigmentosa and other dystrophies. Developments in Ophthalmology. 2010;**47**:160-167

[5] Kalloniatis M, Fletcher EL. Retinitis pigmentosa: Understanding the clinical presentation, mechanisms and treatment options. Clinical and Experimental Optometry. 2004;**87**(2):65-80

[6] Hims MM, Diager SP, Inglehearn CF. Retinitis pigmentosa: Genes, proteins and prospects. Developments in Ophthalmology. 2003;**37**:109-125

[7] Cross N, van Steen C, Zegaoui Y, Satherley A, Angelillo L. Current and future treatment of retinitis Pigmentosa. Clinical Ophthalmology. 2022;**16**:2909-2921

[8] Bok D, Yasumura D, Matthes MT, Ruiz A, Duncan JL, Chappelow AV, et al. Effects of adeno-associated virus-vectored ciliary neurotrophic factor on retinal structure and function in mice with a P216L rds/peripherin mutation. Experimental Eye Research. 2002;**74**(6):719-735

[9] Bush RA, Kononen L, Machida S, Sieving PA. The effect of calcium channel blocker diltiazem on photoreceptor degeneration in the rhodopsin Pro213His rat. Investigative Ophthalmology and Visual Science. 2000;**41**(9):2697-2701

[10] Pawlyk BS, Li T, Scimeca MS, Sandberg MA, Berson EL. Absence of photoreceptor rescue with D-cis-diltiazem in the rd mouse. Investigative Ophthalmology and Visual Science. 2002;**43**(6):1912-1915

[11] Pearce-Kelling SE, Aleman TS, Nickle A, Laties AM, Aguirre GD, Jacobson SG, et al. Calcium channel blocker D-cis-diltiazem does not slow retinal degeneration in the PDE6B mutant rcd1 canine model of retinitis pigmentosa. Molecular Vision. 2001;**7**:42-47

[12] Tao W, Wen R, Goddard MB, Sherman SD, O'Rourke PJ, Stabila PF, et al. Encapsulated cell-based delivery of CNTF reduces photoreceptor degeneration in animal models of retinitis pigmentosa. Investigative Ophthalmology and Visual Science. 2002;**43**(10):3292-3298

[13] Berson EL, Rosner B, Sandberg MA, Hayes KC, Nicholson BW, Weigel-DiFranco C, et al. A randomized trial of vitamin A and vitamin E supplementation for retinitis pigmentosa. Archives of Ophthalmology (Chicago, Ill: 1960). 1993;**111**(6):761-772

[14] Berson EL, Rosner B, Sandberg MA, Weigel-DiFranco C, Moser A, Brockhurst RJ, et al. Clinical

trial of docosahexaenoic acid in patients with retinitis pigmentosa receiving vitamin A treatment. Archives of Ophthalmology (Chicago, Ill: 1960). 2004;**122**(9):1297-1305

[15] Berson EL, Weigel-DiFranco C, Rosner B, Gaudio AR, Sandberg MA. Association of vitamin A supplementation with disease course in children with retinitis pigmentosa. JAMA Ophthalmology. 2018;**136**(5):490-495

[16] Darrow JJ. Luxturna: FDA documents reveal the value of a costly gene therapy. Drug Discovery Today. 2019;**24**(4):949-954

[17] Menghini M, Cehajić-Kapetanovic J, MacLaren RE. Monitoring progression of retinitis pigmentosa: Current recommendations and recent advances. Expert Opinion on Orphan Drugs. 2020;**8**(2-3):67-78. DOI: 10.1080/21678707.2020.1735352

[18] Russell S, Bennett J, Wellman JA, Chung DC, Yu ZF, Tillman A, et al. Efficacy and safety of voretigene neparvovec (AAV2-hRPE65v2) in patients with RPE65-mediated inherited retinal dystrophy: A randomised, controlled, open-label, phase 3 trial. Lancet (London, England). 2017;**390**(10097):849-860

[19] Amato A, Arrigo A, Aragona E, Manitto MP, Saladino A, Bandello F, et al. Gene therapy in inherited retinal diseases: An update on current state of the art. Frontiers in Medicine. 2021;**8**:750586

[20] Battu R, Ratra D, Gopal L. Newer therapeutic options for inherited retinal diseases: Gene and cell replacement therapy. Indian Journal of Ophthalmology. 2022;**70**(7):2316-2325. DOI: 10.4103/ijo.IJO_82_22

[21] Beltran WA, Cideciyan AV, Boye SE, Ye G-J, Iwabe S, Dufour VL, et al. Optimization of retinal gene therapy for X-linked retinitis pigmentosa due to RPGR mutations. Molecular Therapy. 2017;**25**(8):1866-1880

[22] Fischer MD, McClements ME, Martinez-Fernandez de la Camara C, Bellingrath JS, Dauletbekov D, Ramsden SC, et al. Codon-optimized RPGR improves stability and efficacy of AAV8 gene therapy in two mouse models of X-linked retinitis pigmentosa. Molecular Therapy: The Journal of the American Society of Gene Therapy. 2017;**25**(8):1854-1865

[23] Georgiou M, Awadh Hashem S, Daich Varela M, Michaelides M. Gene therapy in X-linked retinitis pigmentosa due to defects in RPGR. International Ophthalmology Clinics. 2021;**61**(4):97-108. DOI: 10.1097/IIO.0000000000000384

[24] Mears AJ, Gieser L, Yan D, Chen C, Fahrner S, Hiriyanna S, et al. Protein-truncation mutations in the RP2 gene in a north American cohort of families with X-linked retinitis pigmentosa. American Journal of Human Genetics. 1999;**64**(3):897-900

[25] Schwahn U, Paland N, Techritz S, Lenzner S, Berger W. Mutations in the X-linked RP2 gene cause intracellular misrouting and loss of the protein. Human Molecular Genetics. 2001;**10**(11):1177-1183

[26] Fahim AT, Sullivan LS, Bowne SJ, Jones KD, Wheaton DKH, Khan NW, et al. X-chromosome inactivation is a biomarker of clinical severity in female carriers of RPGR-associated X-linked retinitis pigmentosa. Ophthalmology Retina. 2020;**4**(5):510-520

[27] Salvetti AP, Nanda A, MacLaren RE. RPGR-related X-linked retinitis pigmentosa carriers with a severe "male pattern". Ophthalmologica

Journal international d'ophtalmologie International journal of ophthalmology Zeitschrift fur Augenheilkunde. 2021;**244**(1):60-67

[28] Aleman TS, Cideciyan AV, Sumaroka A, Schwartz SB, Roman AJ, Windsor EA, et al. Inner retinal abnormalities in X-linked retinitis pigmentosa with RPGR mutations. Investigative Ophthalmology and Visual Science. 2007;**48**(10):4759-4765

[29] Sandberg MA, Rosner B, Weigel-DiFranco C, Dryja TP, Berson EL. Disease course of patients with X-linked retinitis Pigmentosa due to RPGRGene mutations. Investigative Opthalmology and Visual Science. 2007;**48**(3):1298-1304

[30] Vervoort R, Lennon A, Bird AC, Tulloch B, Axton R, Miano MG, et al. Mutational hot spot within a new RPGR exon in X-linked retinitis pigmentosa. Nature Genetics. 2000;**25**(4):462-466

[31] Khanna H, Hurd TW, Lillo C, Shu X, Parapuram SK, He S, et al. RPGR-ORF15, which is mutated in retinitis pigmentosa, associates with SMC1, SMC3, and microtubule transport proteins. Journal of Biological Chemistry. 2005;**280**(39):33580-33587

[32] Rao KN, Li L, Anand M, Khanna H. Ablation of retinal ciliopathy protein RPGR results in altered photoreceptor ciliary composition. Scientific Reports. 2015;**5**(1):11137

[33] Hong DH, Li T. Complex expression pattern of RPGR reveals a role for purine-rich exonic splicing enhancers. Investigative Ophthalmology and Visual Science. 2002;**43**(11):3373-3382

[34] Schlegel J, Hoffmann J, Roll D, Muller B, Gunther S, Zhang W, et al. Toward genome editing in X-linked RP-development of a mouse model with specific treatment relevant features. Translational Research: the Journal of Laboratory and Clinical Medicine. 2019;**203**:57-72

[35] Shu X, Black GC, Rice JM, Hart-Holden N, Jones A, O'Grady A, et al. RPGR mutation analysis and disease: An update. Human Mutation. 2007;**28**(4):322-328

[36] Sun X, Park JH, Gumerson J, Wu Z, Swaroop A, Qian H, et al. Loss of RPGR glutamylation underlies the pathogenic mechanism of retinal dystrophy caused by TTLL5 mutations. Proceedings of the National Academy of Sciences of the United States of America. 2016;**113**(21):E2925-E2934

[37] Cehajic Kapetanovic J, McClements ME, Martinez-Fernandez de la Camara C, MacLaren RE. Molecular strategies for RPGR gene therapy. Genes (Basel). 2019;**10**(9):674

[38] Moreno-Leon L, West EL, O'Hara-Wright M, Li L, Nair R, He J, et al. RPGR isoform imbalance causes ciliary defects due to exon ORF15 mutations in X-linked retinitis pigmentosa (XLRP). Human Molecular Genetics. 2021;**29**(22):3706-3716

[39] Pawlyk BS, Bulgakov OV, Sun X, Adamian M, Shu X, Smith AJ, et al. Photoreceptor rescue by an abbreviated human RPGR gene in a murine model of X-linked retinitis pigmentosa. Gene Therapy. 2016;**23**(2):196-204

[40] Zhang Q, Acland GM, Wu WX, Johnson JL, Pearce-Kelling S, Tulloch B, et al. Different RPGR exon ORF15 mutations in Canids provide insights into photoreceptor cell degeneration. Human Molecular Genetics. 2002;**11**(9):993-1003

[41] Falasconi A, Biagioni M, Novelli E, Piano I, Gargini C, Strettoi E. Retinal

phenotype in the rd9 mutant mouse, a model of X-linked RP. Frontiers in Neuroscience. 2019;**13**(September):991

[42] Thompson DA, Khan NW, Othman MI, Chang B, Jia L, Grahek G, et al. Rd9 is a naturally occurring mouse model of a common form of retinitis pigmentosa caused by mutations in RPGR-ORF15. PLoS One. 2012;**7**(5):e35865

[43] Hong DH, Pawlyk BS, Shang J, Sandberg MA, Berson EL, Li T. A retinitis pigmentosa GTPase regulator (RPGR)-deficient mouse model for X-linked retinitis pigmentosa (RP3). Proceedings of the National Academy of Sciences of the United States of America. 2000;**97**(7):3649-3654

[44] Buck TM, Wijnholds J. Recombinant Adeno-associated viral vectors (rAAV)-vector elements in ocular gene therapy clinical trials and transgene expression and bioactivity assays. International Journal of Molecular Sciences. 2020;**21**(12):4197

[45] Bulcha JT, Wang Y, Ma H, Tai PWL, Gao G. Viral vector platforms within the gene therapy landscape. Signal Transduction and Targeted Therapy. 2021;**6**(1):53

[46] Mendell JR, Al-Zaidy SA, Rodino-Klapac LR, Goodspeed K, Gray SJ, Kay CN, et al. Current clinical applications of In vivo gene therapy with AAVs. Molecular Therapy: the Journal of the American Society of Gene Therapy. 2021;**29**(2):464-488

[47] Issa PC, De Silva SR, Lipinski DM, Singh MS, Mouravlev A, You Q, et al. Assessment of tropism and effectiveness of new primate-derived hybrid recombinant AAV serotypes in the mouse and primate retina. PLoS One. 2013;**8**(4):e60361

[48] Natkunarajah M, Trittibach P, McIntosh J, Duran Y, Barker SE, Smith AJ, et al. Assessment of ocular transduction using single-stranded and self-complementary recombinant adeno-associated virus serotype 2/8. Gene Therapy. 2008;**15**(6):463-467

[49] Burger C, Gorbatyuk OS, Velardo MJ, Peden CS, Williams P, Zolotukhin S, et al. Recombinant AAV viral vectors pseudotyped with viral capsids from serotypes 1, 2, and 5 display differential efficiency and cell tropism after delivery to different regions of the central nervous system. Molecular Therapy: The Journal of the American Society of Gene Therapy. 2004;**10**(2):302-317

[50] Khabou H, Desrosiers M, Winckler C, Fouquet S, Auregan G, Bemelmans AP, et al. Insight into the mechanisms of enhanced retinal transduction by the engineered AAV2 capsid variant -7m8. Biotechnology and Bioengineering. 2016;**113**(12):2712-2724

[51] Ross M, Ofri R. The future of retinal gene therapy: Evolving from subretinal to intravitreal vector delivery. Neural Regeneration Research. 2021;**16**(9):1751-1759

[52] Kong J, Kim SR, Binley K, Pata I, Doi K, Mannik J, et al. Correction of the disease phenotype in the mouse model of stargardt disease by lentiviral gene therapy. Gene Therapy. 2008;**15**(19):1311-1320

[53] Grimm D, Lee JS, Wang L, Desai T, Akache B, Storm TA, et al. In vitro and in vivo gene therapy vector evolution via multispecies interbreeding and retargeting of adeno-associated viruses. Journal of Virology. 2008;**82**(12):5887-5911

[54] Katada Y, Kobayashi K, Tsubota K, Kurihara T. Evaluation of AAV-DJ vector

for retinal gene therapy. Peer Journal. 2019;7:e6317

[55] Covello G, Ibrahim GH, Bacchi N, Casarosa S, Denti MA. Exon skipping through chimeric antisense U1 snRNAs to correct retinitis pigmentosa GTPase-regulator (RPGR) splice defect. Nucleic Acid Therapeutics. 2022;**32**(4):333-349

[56] Gupta A, Kafetzis KN, Tagalakis AD, Yu-Wai-Man C. RNA therapeutics in ophthalmology - Translation to clinical trials. Experimental Eye Research. 2021;**205**:108482

[57] Kuzmin DA, Shutova MV, Johnston NR, Smith OP, Fedorin VV, Kukushkin YS, et al. The clinical landscape for AAV gene therapies. Nature Reviews. Drug Discovery. 2021;**20**(3):173-174

[58] Beltran WA, Cideciyan AV, Lewin AS, Iwabe S, Khanna H, Sumaroka A, et al. Gene therapy rescues photoreceptor blindness in dogs and paves the way for treating human X-linked retinitis pigmentosa. Proceedings of the National Academy of Sciences of the United States of America. 2012;**109**(6):2132-2137

[59] Wu Z, Hiriyanna S, Qian H, Mookherjee S, Campos MM, Gao C, et al. A long-term efficacy study of gene replacement therapy for RPGR-associated retinal degeneration. Human Molecular Genetics. 2015;**24**(14):3956-3970

[60] Song C, Dufour VL, Cideciyan AV, Ye GJ, Swider M, Newmark JA, et al. Dose range finding studies with two RPGR transgenes in a canine model of X-linked retinitis pigmentosa treated with subretinal gene therapy. Human Gene Therapy. 2020;**31**(13-14):743-755

[61] Gumerson JD, Alsufyani A, Yu W, Lei J, Sun X, Dong L, et al. Restoration of RPGR expression in vivo using CRISPR/Cas9 gene editing. Gene Therapy. 2022;**29**(1-2):81-93

[62] Hu S, Du J, Chen N, Jia R, Zhang J, Liu X, et al. In vivo CRISPR/Cas9-mediated genome editing mitigates photoreceptor degeneration in a mouse model of X-linked retinitis pigmentosa. Investigative Ophthalmology and Visual Science. 2020;**61**(4):31

[63] Hong DH, Pawlyk BS, Adamian M, Sandberg MA, Li T. A single, abbreviated RPGR-ORF15 variant reconstitutes RPGR function in vivo. Investigative Ophthalmology and Visual Science. 2005;**46**(2):435-441

[64] Beltran WA, Cideciyan AV, Iwabe S, Lewin AS, Swider M, Guzman JM, et al. Gene therapy for RPGR-XLRP in a canine model results in retained photoreceptors and vision for at least 2.5 years. Investigative Ophthalmology and Visual Science. 2015;**56**(7):2588

[65] Beltran WA, Cideciyan AV, Iwabe S, Swider M, Kosyk MS, McDaid K, et al. Successful arrest of photoreceptor and vision loss expands the therapeutic window of retinal gene therapy to later stages of disease. Proceedings of the National Academy of Sciences of the United States of America. 2015;**112**(43):E5844-E5853

[66] Mookherjee S, Hiriyanna S, Kaneshiro K, Li L, Li Y, Li W, et al. Long-term rescue of cone photoreceptor degeneration in retinitis pigmentosa 2 (RP2)-knockout mice by gene replacement therapy. Human Molecular Genetics. 2015;**24**(22):6446-6458

[67] Deng WT, Dyka FM, Dinculescu A, Li J, Zhu P, Chiodo VA, et al. Stability and safety of an AAV vector for treating RPGR-ORF15 X-linked retinitis pigmentosa. Human Gene Therapy. 2015;**26**(9):593-602

[68] Giacalone JC, Andorf JL, Zhang Q, Burnight ER, Ochoa D, Reutzel AJ, et al. Development of a molecularly stable gene therapy vector for the treatment of RPGR-associated X-linked retinitis pigmentosa. Human Gene Therapy. 2019;**30**(8):967-974

[69] Schlegel J, Hoffmann J, Röll D, Müller B, Günther S, Zhang W, et al. Toward genome editing in X-linked RP-development of a mouse model with specific treatment relevant features. Translational Research. 2019;**203**:57-72

[70] Dufour VL, Cideciyan AV, Ye GJ, Song C, Timmers A, Habecker PL, et al. Toxicity and efficacy evaluation of an adeno-associated virus vector expressing codon-optimized RPGR delivered by subretinal injection in a canine model of X-linked retinitis pigmentosa. Human Gene Therapy. 2020;**31**(3-4):253-267

[71] Michaelides M, Xu J, Wang D, Wong P, Fung A, Forbes A, et al. AAV5-RPGR (botaretigene sparoparvovec) gene therapy for X-linked retinitis pigmentosa (XLRP) demonstrates localized improvements in static perimetry. Investigative Ophthalmology and Visual Science. 2022;**63**(7):3846

[72] Prusky GT, Alam NM, Beekman S, Douglas RM. Rapid quantification of adult and developing mouse spatial vision using a virtual optomotor system. Investigative Ophthalmology and Visual Science. 2004;**45**(12):4611-4616

[73] Tomita H, Sugano E, Fukazawa Y, Isago H, Sugiyama Y, Hiroi T, et al. Visual properties of transgenic rats harboring the channelrhodopsin-2 gene regulated by the thy-1.2 promoter. PLoS One. 2009;**4**(11):e7679

[74] Gundogan FC, Tas A, Sobaci G. Electroretinogram in hereditary retinal disorders. In: Electroretinograms. 1st ed. IntechOpen; 2011. pp. 95-132. DOI: 10.5772/21704

[75] Miyake Y, Shinoda K. Clinical electrophysiology. In: Ryan SJ, Sadda SR, Hinton DR, Schachat AP, Sadda SR, Wilkinson CP, et al., editors. Retina. London: W.B. Saunders; 2013. pp. 202-226

[76] Robson AG, Frishman LJ, Grigg J, Hamilton R, Jeffrey BG, Kondo M, et al. ISCEV standard for full-field clinical electroretinography (2022 update). Documenta Ophthalmologica Advances in Ophthalmology. 2022;**144**(3):165-177

[77] Benchorin G, Calton MA, Beaulieu MO, Vollrath D. Assessment of murine retinal function by Electroretinography. Bio-Protocol. 2017;**7**(7):e2218

[78] Kinoshita J, Peachey NS. Noninvasive electroretinographic procedures for the study of the mouse retina. Current Protocols in Mouse Biology. 2018;**8**(1):1-16

[79] Pinto LH, Invergo B, Shimomura K, Takahashi JS, Troy JB. Interpretation of the mouse electroretinogram. Documenta Ophthalmologica Advances in Ophthalmology. 2007;**115**(3):127-136

[80] Janaky M, Palffy A, Horvath G, Tuboly G, Benedek G. Pattern-reversal electroretinograms and visual evoked potentials in retinitis pigmentosa. Documenta Ophthalmologica Advances in Ophthalmology. 2008;**117**(1):27-36

[81] Marenna S, Castoldi V, d'Isa R, Marco C, Comi G, Leocani L. Semi-invasive and non-invasive recording of visual evoked potentials in mice. Documenta Ophthalmologica Advances in Ophthalmology. 2019;**138**(3):169-179

[82] Ridder WH 3rd, Nusinowitz S. The visual evoked potential in the mouse--origins and response characteristics. Vision Research. 2006;**46**(6-7):902-913

[83] Tomiyama Y, Fujita K, Nishiguchi KM, Tokashiki N, Daigaku R, Tabata K, et al. Measurement of electroretinograms and visually evoked potentials in awake moving mice. PLoS One. 2016;**11**(6):e0156927

[84] Handley SE, Šuštar M, Tekavčič PM. What can visual electrophysiology tell about possible visual-field defects in paediatric patients. Eye. 2021;**35**(9):2354-2373

[85] Drexler W, Sattmann H, Hermann B, Ko TH, Stur M, Unterhuber A, et al. Enhanced visualization of macular pathology with the use of ultrahigh-resolution optical coherence tomography. Archives of Ophthalmology (Chicago, Ill: 1960). 2003;**121**(5):695-706

[86] Battaglia Parodi M, La Spina C, Triolo G, Riccieri F, Pierro L, Gagliardi M, et al. Correlation of SD-OCT findings and visual function in patients with retinitis pigmentosa. Graefe's Archive for Clinical and Experimental Ophthalmology = Albrecht von Graefes Archiv fur klinische und experimentelle Ophthalmologie. 2016;**254**(7):1275-1279

[87] Cai CX, Locke KG, Ramachandran R, Birch DG, Hood DC. A comparison of progressive loss of the ellipsoid zone (EZ) band in autosomal dominant and x-linked retinitis pigmentosa. Investigative Ophthalmology and Visual Science. 2014;**55**(11):7417-7422

[88] Fischer MD, Fleischhauer JC, Gillies MC, Sutter FK, Helbig H, Barthelmes D. A new method to monitor visual field defects caused by photoreceptor degeneration by quantitative optical coherence tomography. Investigative Ophthalmology and Visual Science. 2008;**49**(8):3617-3621

[89] Hood DC, Ramachandran R, Holopigian K, Lazow M, Birch DG, Greenstein VC. Method for deriving visual field boundaries from OCT scans of patients with retinitis pigmentosa. Biomedical Optics Express. 2011;**2**(5):1106-1114

[90] Menghini M, Lujan BJ, Zayit-Soudry S, Syed R, Porco TC, Bayabo K, et al. Correlation of outer nuclear layer thickness with cone density values in patients with retinitis pigmentosa and healthy subjects. Investigative Ophthalmology and Visual Science. 2014;**56**(1):372-381

[91] Sousa K, Fernandes T, Gentil R, Mendonca L, Falcao M. Outer retinal layers as predictors of visual acuity in retinitis pigmentosa: A cross-sectional study. Graefe's Archive for Clinical and Experimental Ophthalmology = Albrecht von Graefes Archiv fur klinische und experimentelle Ophthalmologie. 2019;**257**(2):265-271

[92] Nakazawa M, Hara A, Ishiguro SI. Optical coherence tomography of animal models of retinitis pigmentosa: From animal studies to clinical applications. BioMed Research International. 2019;**2019**:8276140

[93] Barone I, Novelli E, Piano I, Gargini C, Strettoi E. Environmental enrichment extends photoreceptor survival and visual function in a mouse model of retinitis pigmentosa. PLoS One. 2012;**7**(11):e50726

[94] Shintani K, Shechtman DL, Gurwood AS. Review and update: Current treatment trends for patients

with retinitis pigmentosa. Optometry. 2009;**80**(7):384-401

[95] Hong Y, Li H, Sun Y, Ji Y. A review of complicated cataract in retinitis pigmentosa: Pathogenesis and cataract surgery. Journal of Ophthalmology. 2020;**2020**:6699103

[96] Winkler PA, Occelli LM, Petersen-Jones SM. Large animal models of inherited retinal degenerations: A review. Cells. 2020;**9**(4):882. DOI: 10.3390/cells9040882

[97] Martinez-Fernandez De La Camara C, Cehajic-Kapetanovic J, MacLaren RE. RPGR gene therapy presents challenges in cloning the coding sequence. Expert Opinion on Biological Therapy. 2020;**20**(1):63-71. DOI: 10.1080/14712598.2020.1680635

[98] Peng Y, Tang L, Zhou Y. Subretinal injection: A review on the novel route of therapeutic delivery for vitreoretinal diseases. Ophthalmic Research. 2017;**58**(4):217-226

[99] Qi Y, Dai X, Zhang H, He Y, Zhang Y, Han J, et al. Trans-corneal subretinal injection in mice and its effect on the function and morphology of the retina. PLoS One. 2015;**10**(8):e0136523

[100] Weng CY. Bilateral subretinal voretigene neparvovec-rzyl (luxturna) gene therapy. Ophthalmology Retina. 2019;**3**(5):450

[101] De Silva SR, Charbel Issa P, Singh MS, Lipinski DM, Barnea-Cramer AO, Walker NJ, et al. Single residue AAV capsid mutation improves transduction of photoreceptors in the Abca4(−/−) mouse and bipolar cells in the rd1 mouse and human retina ex vivo. Gene Therapy. 2016;**23**(11):767-774

[102] Stout JT, Francis PJ. Surgical approaches to gene and stem cell therapy for retinal disease. Human Gene Therapy. 2011;**22**(5):531-535

[103] Datta P, Ruffcorn A, Seo S. Limited time window for retinal gene therapy in a preclinical model of ciliopathy. Human Molecular Genetics. 2020;**29**(14):2337-2352

[104] Mansouri V. X-linked retinitis pigmentosa gene therapy: Preclinical aspects. Ophthalmology and Therapy. 2023;**12**(1):7-34

[105] [Creative Commons License]: Attribution-NonCommercial 4.0 International. Available from: http://creativecommons.org/licenses/by-nc/4.0/ [Accessed: August 23, 2024]

Chapter 5

Newer Medical Management Options in Glaucoma

Sangeetha Sreenivasa Pai

Abstract

Glaucoma is a progressive optic neuropathy and the only risk factor which can be controlled in order to stabilise glaucoma is intraocular pressure. We are all aware of the conventional eye drops used to reduce intraocular pressures in glaucoma, however, recently, some new medications and devices have been developed. This chapter will give an insight in to the time line of existing glaucoma eye drops, the problems associated with them and the need to have newer medications. I have described two newer medications in detail and have also written about some implants which are in the phase of development.

Keywords: glaucoma, Roclanda, ROCK inhibitor, ROCK, OMDI, PAP, glaucoma implants

1. Introduction

Glaucoma, as we know, is a chronic, progressive eye disease, which leads to optic neuropathy and visual field loss. A lot of advances have happened in pharmacotherapy of glaucoma over the years; however, recently, there has been a rise in the number of newer medications and devices that control intraocular pressures (IOP) which help stabilise glaucoma thereby avoiding the need for surgical management. They also aim to improve patient compliance, reduce ocular and systemic side effects and provide more effective long term pressure control. The newer agents that we are going to discuss here are Rho kinase inhibitors, OMDI and some newer implants.

1.1 Timeline of glaucoma eye drops

See **Figure 1**.

We have these five classes of anti-glaucoma medications; however, there are a lot of issues encountered in clinical practice with them [1].

They are:

1. Intolerance to the side effects of these eye drops, allergy to eye drops or contra-indications to the medications.

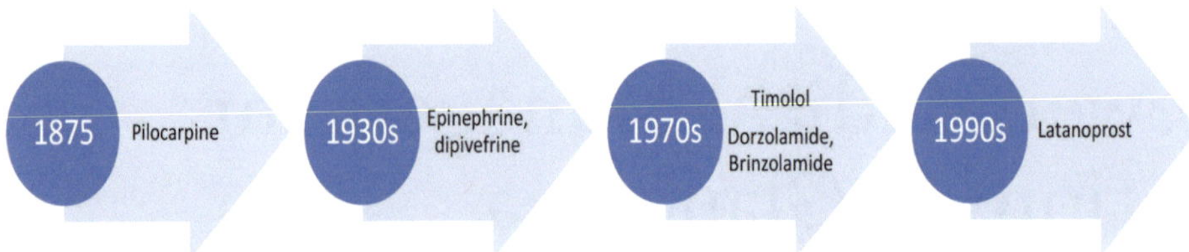

Figure 1.
Timeline of glaucoma eye drops [1].

2. IOP lowering insufficient on maximum medications demanding the need for surgery with its own short- and long-term complications.

3. Compliance issues to multiple eye drops.

The other treatment option available is lasers like selective laser trabeculoplasty (SLT) which acts on trabecular meshwork; however, it is not effective in all types of glaucoma.

Also, as a matter of fact, none of the available medications target the underlying cause of elevated IOP which increases outflow resistance in trabecular meshwork.

In short, there is an unmet need to have other medical management options for glaucoma with same/improved efficacy and better adverse effect profile.

I propose that an ideal medication for glaucoma should be:

a. Highly effective during diurnal and nocturnal period

b. Easy to use, once a day dosing which will improve compliance

c. Well tolerated with the minimal adverse effects

d. Neuroprotective activity and improved ocular perfusion would be desirable.

1.2 The evolution of ROCK inhibitors

Let us discuss the physiology of aqueous humour secretion and outflow first before going deeper into ROCK inhibitors.

There are 3 steps involved in aqueous humour production. They are passive diffusion, ultrafiltration and active secretion. About 85–90% of the drainage occurs through trabecular meshwork which is the conventional outflow pathway [2]. The rest of the outflow occurs *via* the uveoscleral route which is also called the non-conventional pathway [3].

1.3 What is ROCK, Rho-associated protein kinase?

Rho kinase (effector protein) attaches to Rho which is a molecular switch inside the cells to form ROCK. This ROCK (complex Rho- associated coiled- coil containing protein kinase) modifies Rho through a cascade of intra-cellular changes thereby regulating various physiological processes in our body [4, 5]. The ROCK also plays a role in cellular adhesions and stiffening and also reorganises extracellular matrix due to its effect on actomyosin contractile forces [6]. These factors determine aqueous outflow through the trabecular meshwork pathway, thus proving that rho kinase mechanism has a direct relationship to the normal aqueous outflow through conventional route.

In 2014, ROCK inhibitors (ripasudil) were approved in Japan for the treatment of primary open-angle glaucoma (POAG) and ocular hypertension (OHT) [1]. The role of ROCK inhibitors is now being explored in other ocular conditions such as Fuchs dystrophy, cataract, age-related macular degeneration and proliferative vitreous retinopathy.

1.4 Mechanism of action of ROCK inhibitors

a. Relaxes trabecular meshwork smooth muscle cells

b. Improves Schlemm's canal (SC) cell elasticity, thereby decrease funnelling effect

c. Improves blood flow (vascular smooth muscle relaxation), thereby decreasing EVP.

ROCK causes TM contraction resulting in the formation of CLANs, thereby increasing outflow resistance [6]. It is shown that ROCK inhibitors decrease the density of actin stress fibres (less CLANs—cross-linked Actin Networks) causing TM cells to relax.

1.5 Other mechanisms

It is also found that ROCK inhibitors have effect on ECM synthesis, thereby reducing IOP by ECM remodelling [7]. It also reduces episcleral venous pressure. In addition to this, it is found that ROCK inhibitors also have a neuro-protective effect as it increases the blood supply of optic nerve due to vasodilatory properties as well as act as a free radical scavenger in TM.

The role of ROCK inhibitors in limiting tissue fibrosis is also being studied in animals [8]. Further studies in humans are required to determine safety and efficacy.

Some of the ROCK inhibitors that are studied are (**Table 1**).

Ripasudil was the first ROCK inhibitor, which was approved in Japan for the treatment of glaucoma and OHT in 2014. Trials also studied combinations with Timolol 0.5% BD and Latanoprost 0.005% OD, and it was seen that a greater IOP reduction was possible when combined with Timolol [9].

1.6 Netarsudil (AR-13324): (Rhopressa, Rhokiinsa)

It has dual action as it is a Rho kinase inhibitor as well as norepinephrine transport inhibitor. It was approved for use in US to treat glaucoma in 2017. It decreases aqueous humour production and decreases episcleral venous pressure [10–12].

ROCKET 1 and 2 trials compared Netarsudil 0.02% OD and BD formulations to Timolol 0.5% BD in patients with ocular hypertension and open-angle glaucoma [13]. Netarsudil was non-inferior to timolol in all these studies. Conjunctival hyperemia was reported in 50–53% of patients for Netarsudil OD and 59% for Netarsudil BD, compared to only 8–10% for timolol. Conjunctival haemorrhage was reported in 13.3–15%, 17% and 0% of patients in the Netarsudil OD, Netarsudil BD and Timolol groups, respectively.

Drug	SNJ-1656 (Y-39983)	AR-12286	Ripasudil (K-115)	Netarsudil (AR-13324, Rhopressa, Rhokiinsa)
IOP reduction	3 + 1.2 mm Hg	7 mmm Hg	2–4.4 mm Hg	5.5 mm Hg with 0.01% 5.7 mm Hg with 0.02% and 6.8 mm Hg with 0.005% latanoprost
Percentage of drug	0.1%	0.5%	0.4%	0.01%, 0.02%
Dosing	OD or BD	OD or BD	BD	OD
Adverse effects	Conjunctival hyperemia 100%	Conjunctival hyperemia 60%, irritation, lacrimation, blurred vision	Conjunctival hyperemia 70%, blepharitis, allergic conjunctivitis	Conjunctival hyperemia—mild in 52%, 57% and 15%, respectively, lacrimation (6%), sub-conjunctival haemorrhage (5%)

Table 1.
Table showing ROCK inhibitors [1].

The conjunctival haemorrhages seen in these studies were small, peri-limbal microhemorrhages [13]. Another adverse effect noted was the appearance of cornea verticillata which was observed more in the Netarsudil cohort than the Timolol cohort, and this was very much similar to the Amiodarone-related verticillata [14]. Visual acuity was not affected by any of these side effects, and resolution occurred after cessation of netarsudil.

The efficacy of fixed-dose combinations of Netarsudil 0.01% and 0.02% with Latanoprost 0.005% was also studied, and it was found that Netarsudil 0.02% with Latanoprost 0.005% was superior than each of the medication alone or the combination with 0.01% [15].

MERCURY-3 trial was a non-inferiority study done to compare Roclanda (Latanoprost 0.005% + Netarsudil 0.02%) with the FDC commonly used which was Ganfort in patients with open-angle glaucoma and ocular hypertension. It was concluded that once daily Roclanda was non-inferior to Ganfort in terms of IOP reduction. Roclanda (Santen) has been launched in the UK in 2024 and is approved by NICE. It is a fixed-dose combination of Netarsudil 0.02% and Latanoprost 0.005%, to be used once a day in the evening.

1.7 Adverse reactions of Roclanda

a. Conjunctival hyperemia:

Conjunctival hyperaemia was the most frequently reported side effect due to the vasodilatory effect. It was mild in the majority of cases. Very small percentage of people had moderate-to-severe hyperemia which led to discontinuation of drug (5.0% in Phase 3 clinical studies) [16].

b. Cornea verticillata:

The incidence was 11% in phase 3 studies; it did not affect vision and settled after discontinuation of the drug. Some were at higher risk than the others such as elderly, males and white ethnicity.

c. Iris pigmentation:

This was due to the Latanoprost present in the combination.

In my limited clinical experience with Roclanda, I can say that it has had varied adverse effect profile. It is well tolerated by 70–80% of the patients, whereas the drug had to be discontinued in the remaining 20–30% due to severe sub-conjunctival haemorrhage and cosmetic issues associated with it.

1.8 Effects of ROCK inhibitors on conjunctival scarring after glaucoma surgery

As we all know, the most common cause for the failure of glaucoma filtration surgery is the formation of excessive subconjunctival fibrosis which prevents or limits the egress of aqueous humour [17]. TGF-beta is an important cytokine involved in post-operative wound healing and scar formation. Animal studies have showed that treatment with Y-27632 and Ripasudil leads to inhibition of TGF-beta and alpha SMA, thereby decreasing the scarring of blebs [18, 19]. This mechanism of ROCK inhibitors is yet to be studied in humans, and if proved useful, it will improve the post-operative outcomes significantly.

1.9 Conclusion

As we can see, Rho kinase (ROCK) inhibitors represent a significant development in the pharmacological management of glaucoma. By targeting the Rho kinase pathway, these medications effectively reduce intraocular pressure through dual mechanism of action. It is a new drug combination, and therefore, there will be some stigma associated with its use. However, I believe with time Roclanda will emerge as an effective alternative in the arsenal of medical options for glaucoma management, especially in patients with multiple drug allergies and elderly patients not keen on surgery.

2. OMDI

The second newer medication that we are going to discuss in this chapter is Omidenepeg Isopropyl (OMDI).

As we know that 1990s saw the introduction of PG analogues. Today, we know four different medications in this class which are Latanoprost, Tafluprost, Travoprost and Bimatoprost. They are often prescribed as the first-line treatment for glaucoma according to NICE guidelines as they have the highest intraocular pressure reduction (25–30%), suppression of diurnal variation of intraocular pressure, effectiveness in all types of glaucoma, additive effects with other medications, good safety profile and good compliance due to once daily dosing. Despite this, there are some concerns with these medications. They are as follows:

Prostaglandin-associated periorbitopathy (PAP):

a. The long-term usage of PG analogues causes local side effects such as hyperpigmentation of iris and eyelids, hypertrichiasis, lengthening of lashes, involution of blepharochalasis, periorbital fat loss, enophthalmos, deepening of upper eyelid sulcus (DUES), hardening of eyelids and ptosis. This constellation of findings has been called prostaglandin associated periorbitopathy or PAP. These local changes can affect the adherence to medication regime due to cosmetic concerns, result in erroneous IOP readings and can cause surgical failures [20–22].

A small number of patients are non/poor responders to prostaglandin analogues (< 10–15% IOP reduction).

b. So, we are in need of an alternative, which is as effective and tolerable as PG analogues with less side effects to treat the non-responders and patients with PAP [23].

It has been found that the E-prostanoid (EP) subtype 1–4 receptors for PGE2 also play an important role in IOP regulation especially the E-prostanoid receptor 2 (EP2) in addition to the FP receptors [24]. OMDI 0.002% was the first approved EP2 receptor agonist formulation approved in Japan to be used as IOP-reducing agent [25].

OMDI has also showed non-inferiority with Latanoprost in studies [26]. OMDI is currently also approved in most of the Eastern countries [20].

2.1 Pharmacological profile

OMDI is a prodrug and is hydrolysed to OMD Omidenepeg which is the active form and is a highly selective EP2 receptor agonist with minimal to no detectable effects on other prostanoid receptors [22, 27]. Therefore, PAP (which happens due to nonspecific binding to FP receptor) does not occur. It has also been shown that OMDI does not cause deepening of upper eyelid sulcus because of its varied effect on ECM [20].

2.2 Mechanism of action

OMDI is an EP2 receptor (present in ciliary body and TM) agonist, which means it increases both trabecular and uveoscleral outflow through G protein-mediated signalling pathways [27].

Various trials were done to study the efficacy of OMDI. Some of them were AYAME, RENGE, FUGI, SPECTRUM and so on where OMDI was tested against Latanoprost, combination with Timolol and in non-responders to Latanoprost, respectively [20]. It was concluded that OMDI 0.002% was very effective as once a day dosing in glaucoma and OHT [21, 28, 29].

2.3 Adverse effects

The side effect noted was again similar to ROCK inhibitors which was conjunctival hyperemia 19.7%. There were some instances of corneal thickening and macular oedema as well [20].

Conjunctival hyperemia is very common and milder than ROCK inhibitors and resolves fast [30]. Also, the average increase in corneal thickness was not clinically significant to affect IOP readings. However, caution is recommended in pseudophakes and aphakes because RENGE study showed that the incidence of macular oedema in pseudophakes was almost 50% and also in patients with iritis or uveitis because of the increased risk of cystoid macular oedema [31].

2.4 Contraindications

OMDI is contraindicated in cases of allergy and also along with PG analogues [32]. There are no clinical reports of its concomitant effect with other glaucoma eye drops except Timolol, so caution is recommended until the safety has been confirmed [32].

2.5 Conclusion

Therefore, I can conclude that OMDI is yet another very effective agent available to be used in glaucoma patients, and the advantage being it has double action, it can even be employed as first-line treatment. Studies have shown good adherence to the once daily dosing regimen and better safety profile with little or no PAP. It is already used in the Eastern countries but is not yet available for use in the UK. I hope OMDI will emerge as a useful alternative in the list of glaucoma medications in the future but with caution in pseudophakes and aphakes. With more research, hopefully, the additive effects along with other glaucoma medications will be clearer.

3. Other drugs in the pipeline

NCX 470 (Nicox SA): This is a PGA formed from nitric oxide donating compound useful in glaucoma and OHT in animal studies [33]. This is a nitric oxide donating prostaglandin analogue similar to Vyzulta.

Cromakalim prodrug (CKLP1): This is an ATP-sensitive potassium channel opener which decreases EVP, thereby reducing IOP significantly in animal studies [34].

QLS-101 (Qlaris Bio): This is yet another ATP-sensitive potassium channel opener aimed to reduce EVP [35].

3.1 Sustained drug delivery systems: Durysta (Allergan)

This is a rod-shaped, biodegradable polymer matrix containing 10 μm of Bimatoprost and was approved in 2020. It is inserted in to the iridocorneal angle in an outpatient basis, and it releases the drug steadily for 3–4 months or sometimes longer eliminating the need for removal. Some studies have shown concerns regarding corneal endothelial loss with these implants [36, 37].

3.2 The iDose implant (Glaukos)

This is a Titanium implant with a scleral anchor, and it releases Travoprost into the anterior chamber. The effect would last 6–12 months. Unlike Durysta, this implant needs to be removed and replaced with a new device once the drug has been completely released. Intraoperative gonioscopy with visualisation of TM and accuracy of placement in TM is very important to achieve the satisfactory results.

3.3 OTX-TIC intracameral implant

This is a soft hydrogel containing Travoprost-loaded micro particles. After injecting in to the angle, the meshwork gets hydrated which lead to the diffusion of the drug particles.

3.4 Travoprost XR

Another rod-shaped intracameral implant which releases Travoprost for 6–12 months, and it uses nanoparticles. Originally created by Envisia Therapeutics, the system is now being developed by Aerie/Alcon [38].

3.5 Latanoprost FA SR

It is yet another intracameral implant being studied which will deliver Latanoprost. It is currently in Phase II studies [38].

3.6 IOL-haptic-based drug delivery

This is basically a hydrophobic IOL with the drug pads at optic haptic junction, injected in the capsular bag through cataract surgery incision, and the drug is released into the aqueous humour for up to three years [38].

3.7 Bimatoprost ring

This is a ring-shaped Bimatoprost implant covered with silicone matrix and an inner poly(propylene) core for structural support. The diameter of the ring ranges from 24 mm to 29 mm. The device is inserted between the upper and lower fornix and is replaced after six months, and it can be done as an outpatient procedure.

3.8 Vyzulta

Latanoprostene bunod 0.024% (LBN, Vyzulta) releases nitric oxide in addition to Latanoprost, thereby relaxing the TM and Schlemm's canal and improving outflow. Some adverse effects were noted in trials such as conjunctival hyperemia and irritation [39].

3.9 Drug-free, non-surgical treatment

This strategy is being explored in animal studies. It involves expanding the suprachoroidal space (SCS) of the eye with an *in situ*-forming hydrogel injected using a microneedle, and it has showed consistent IOP reduction in animals up to 4 months.

4. Conclusion

All these newer implants look very effective, compliant and can replace traditional eye drops in the future. But the availability and access to such implants is still questionable, especially in the underdeveloped countries [40].

Abbreviations

IOP	intraocular pressure
TM	trabecular meshwork
SC	Schlemm's canal

PGA	prostaglandin analogues
AH	aqueous humour
IOL	intraocular lens
EVP	episcleral venous pressure
OHT	ocular hypertension
FDC	fixed-dose combination

Author details

Sangeetha Sreenivasa Pai
Yeovil District Hospital, Somerset NHS Foundation Trust, United Kingdom

*Address all correspondence to: sanvij87@gmail.com

References

[1] Tanna AP, Johnson M. Rho kinase inhibitors as a novel treatment for glaucoma and ocular hypertension. Ophthalmology. 2018;**125**(11):1741-1756

[2] Tamm ER. The trabecular meshwork outflow pathways: Structural and functional aspects. Experimental Eye Research. 2009;**88**(4):648-655

[3] Bill A, Phillips CI. Uveoscleral drainage of aqueous humor in human eyes. Experimental Eye Research. 1971;**12**(3):275-281

[4] Narayan R. We will 'ROCK' you? The role of Rho kinase inhibitors in eye care. Optician. 2020;**2020**(1):8191-1

[5] Berrino E, Supuran CT. Rho-kinase inhibitors in the management of glaucoma. Expert Opinion on Therapeutic Patents. 2019;**29**(10):817-827

[6] Moura-Coelho N, Tavares Ferreira J, Bruxelas CP, Dutra-Medeiros M, Cunha JP, Pinto Proença R. Rho kinase inhibitors-a review on the physiology and clinical use in ophthalmology. Graefe's Archive for Clinical and Experimental Ophthalmology. Jun 2019;**257**(6):1101-1117. DOI: 10.1007/s00417-019-04283-5. Epub 2019 Mar 7

[7] Honjo M, Tanihara H. Impact of the clinical use of ROCK inhibitor on the pathogenesis and treatment of glaucoma. The Japanese Journal of Ophthalmology. 2018;**62**(2):109-126

[8] Aziz M, Kuchtey RW. The trabecular meshwork and ROCK inhibitors-reviewing the mechanisms behind one of the newest classes of glaucoma drugs. Glaucoma Today. May/June 2019

[9] Tanihara H, Inoue T, Yamamoto T, et al. Additive intraocular pressure-lowering effects of the rho kinase inhibitor Ripasudil (K-115) combined with Timolol or Latanoprost: A report of 2 randomized clinical trials. JAMA Ophthalmology. 2015;**133**(7):755-761

[10] Wang RF, Williamson JE, Kopczynski C, Serle JB. Effect of 0. 04% AR-13324, a ROCK, and norepinephrine transporter inhibitor, on aqueous humor dynamics in normotensive monkey eyes. Journal of Glaucoma. 2015;**24**(1):51-54

[11] Li G, Mukherjee D, Navarro I, et al. Visualization of conventional outflow tissue responses to netarsudil in living mouse eyes. European Journal of Pharmacology. 2016;**787**:20-31

[12] Bacharach J, Dubiner HB, Levy B, et al. Double-masked, randomized, dose-response study of AR-13324 versus latanoprost in patients with elevated intraocular pressure. Ophthalmology. 2015;**122**(2):302-307

[13] Serle JB, Katz LJ, McLaurin E, Heah T, Ramirez-Davis N, Usner DW, et al. Two phase 3 clinical trials comparing the safety and efficacy of netarsudil to timolol in patients with elevated intraocular pressure: Rho Kinase Elevated IOP Treatment Trial 1 and 2 (ROCKET-1 and ROCKET-2). American Journal of Ophthalmology. Feb 2018;**186**:116-127. DOI: 10.1016/j.ajo.2017.11.019. Epub 2017 Dec 1

[14] Aerie Pharmaceuticals, Inc. Presentation Regarding Rhopressa to Dermatologic and Ophthalmic Drugs Advisory Committee of the United States Food and Drug Administration. Administration US Food and Drug Administration, ed. 2017

[15] Lewis RA, Levy B, Ramirez N, et al. Fixed-dose combination of AR-13324 and latanoprost: A double-masked, 28-day, randomised, controlled study in patients with open-angle glaucoma or ocular hypertension. The British Journal of Ophthalmology. 2016;**100**(3):339-344

[16] Stalmans I, Lim KS, Oddone F, Fichtl M, Belda JI, Hommer A, et al. MERCURY-3: A randomized comparison of netarsudil/latanoprost and bimatoprost/timolol in open-angle glaucoma and ocular hypertension. Graefe's Archive for Clinical and Experimental Ophthalmology. 2024;**262**(1):179-190. DOI: 10.1007/s00417-023-06192-0. Epub 2023 Aug 24

[17] Skuta GL, Parrish RK. 2nd wound healing in glaucoma filtering surgery. Survey of Ophthalmology. 1987;**32**(3):149-170

[18] Honjo M, Tanihara H, Kameda T, Kawaji T, Yoshimura N, Araie M. Potential role of Rho-associated protein kinase inhibitor Y-27632 in glaucoma filtration surgery. Investigative Ophthalmology and Visual Science. Dec 2007;**48**(12):5549-5557. DOI: 10.1167/iovs.07-0878

[19] Van de Velde S, Van Bergen T, Vandewalle E, et al. Rho kinase inhibitor AMA0526 improves surgical outcome in a rabbit model of glaucoma filtration surgery. Progress in Brain Research. 2015;**220**:283-297

[20] Matsuo M, Matsuoka Y, Tanito M. Efficacy and patient tolerability of Omidenepag isopropyl in the treatment of glaucoma and ocular hypertension. Clinical Ophthalmology. 2022;**16**:1261-1279. DOI: 10.2147/OPTH.S340386

[21] Aihara M. Prostanoid receptor agonists for glaucoma treatment. Japanese Journal of Ophthalmology. 2021;**65**(5):581-590. DOI: 10.1007/s10384-021-00844-6

[22] Tanito M, Ishida A, Ichioka S, et al. Proposal of a simple grading system integrating cosmetic and tonometric aspects of prostaglandin-associated periorbitopathy. Medicine. 2021;**100**(34):e26874. DOI: 10.1097/MD.0000000000026874

[23] Ikeda Y, Mori K, Ishibashi T, Naruse S, Nakajima N, Kinoshita S. Latanoprost nonresponders with open-angle glaucoma in the Japanese population. Japanese Journal of Ophthalmology. 2006;**50**(2):153-157. DOI: 10.1007/s10384-005-0293-x

[24] Saeki T, Ota T, Aihara M, Araie M. Effects of prostanoid EP agonists on mouse intraocular pressure. Investigative Ophthalmology & Visual Science. 2009;**50**(5):2201-2208. DOI: 10.1167/iovs.08-2800

[25] Iwamura R, Tanaka M, Okanari E, et al. Identification of a selective, non-prostanoid EP2 receptor agonist for the treatment of glaucoma: Omidenepag and its prodrug omidenepag isopropyl. Journal of Medicinal Chemistry. 2018;**61**(15):6869-6891. DOI: 10.1021/acs.jmedchem.8b00808

[26] Aihara M, Lu F, Kawata H, Iwata A, Odani-Kawabata N, Shams NK. Omidenepag isopropyl versus latanoprost in primary open-angle glaucoma and ocular hypertension: The phase 3 AYAME study. American Journal of Ophthalmology. 2020;**220**:53-63. DOI: 10.1016/j.ajo.2020.06.003

[27] Kirihara T, Taniguchi T, Yamamura K, et al. Pharmacologic characterization of omidenepag isopropyl, a novel selective EP2 receptor agonist, as an

ocular hypotensive agent. Investigative Ophthalmology & Visual Science. 2018;**59**(1):145-153. DOI: 10.1167/iovs.17-22745

[28] Miki A, Miyamoto E, Ishida N, Shii D, Hori K, LESPOIR Research Group. Efficacy and safety of Omidenepag isopropyl 0.002% ophthalmic solution: A retrospective analysis of real-world data in Japan. Advances in Therapy. 2022;**39**(5):2085-2095. DOI: 10.1007/s12325-022-02069-6. Epub 2022 Mar 14

[29] Shiratori N, Nishio Y, Takeda A, et al. Twenty-four-hour intraocular pressure control with omidenepag isopropyl 0.002% in patients with glaucoma and ocular hypertension. Clinical Ophthalmology. 2021;**15**:3997-4003. DOI: 10.2147/OPTH.S333042

[30] Terao E, Nakakura S, Fujisawa Y, et al. Time course of conjunctival hyperemia induced by omidenepag isopropyl ophthalmic solution 0.002%: A pilot, comparative study versus ripasudil 0.4. BMJ Open Ophthalmology. 2020;**5**(1):e000538. DOI: 10.1136/bmjophth-2020-000538

[31] Aihara M, Lu F, Kawata H, Iwata A, Odani-Kawabata N. Twelve-month efficacy and safety of omidenepag isopropyl, a selective EP2 agonist, in open-angle glaucoma and ocular hypertension: The RENGE study. Japanese Journal of Ophthalmology. 2021;**65**:810-819. DOI: 10.1007/s10384-021-00868-y

[32] Santen Pharmaceutical. EYBELIS ophthalmic solution 0.002%: prescribing information [Japanese]; 2018. Available from: https://www.santen.co.jp/medical-channel/di/tenpu/DD067_eybelis.pdf

[33] Impagnatiello F, Bastia E, Almirante N, et al. Prostaglandin analogues and nitric oxide contribution in the treatment of ocular hypertension and glaucoma. British Journal of Pharmacology. 2019;**176**(8):1079-1089

[34] Roy Chowdhury U, Kudgus RA, Holman BH, et al. Pharmacological profile and ocular hypotensive effects of cromakalim prodrug 1, a novel atp-sensitive potassium channel opener, in normotensive dogs and nonhuman primates. Journal of Ocular Pharmacology and Therapeutics. 2021;**37**(5):251-260

[35] Spiegle L. The glaucoma medication pipeline. Review of Ophthalmology. 10 May 2022

[36] Shirley M. Bimatoprost implant: First approval. Drugs & Aging. 2020;**37**(6):457-462

[37] Medeiros FA, Sheybani A, Shah MM, et al. Single administration of intracameral bimatoprost implant 10 microg in patients with open-angle glaucoma or ocular hypertension. Ophthalmology and Therapy. 2022;**11**(4):1517-1537

[38] Kent C. Sustained delivery and glaucoma: An update. Review of Ophthalmology. 10 Jan 2023

[39] Clinical Review Report: Latanoprostene Bunod (Vyzulta): (Bausch Health, Canada Inc.): Indication: For the Reduction of Intraocular Pressure (IOP) in Patients with Open-Angle Glaucoma or Ocular Hypertension [Internet]. Ottawa (ON): Canadian Agency for Drugs and Technologies in Health; 2019. Discussion. Available from: https://www.ncbi.nlm.nih.gov/books/NBK549667/

[40] Chae JJ, Jung JH, Zhu W, Gerberich BG, Bahrani Fard MR, Grossniklaus HE, et al. Drug-free, nonsurgical reduction of intraocular pressure for four months after Suprachoroidal injection of hyaluronic acid hydrogel. Advanced Science (Weinh). 2020;**8**(2):2001908. DOI: 10.1002/advs.202001908

Chapter 6

Exosomes and Exosome-Derived miRNAs: Current Knowledge and Future Aspects

Ke Mao

Abstract

In this chapter, we mainly discuss exosome-derived miRNAs in diagnosis and therapy of common ocular diseases, since dysregulation of exosomes and their miRNA cargo is believed to be correlated to vision blur. First, we introduce the origin of exosomes and exosome-derived miRNAs. Next, we summarize identified miRNAs and their pathogenic mechanisms to common ophthalmic diseases. Finally, we discuss the potential roles of exosomes and miRNAs in diagnosis and therapeutic treatments in future clinical applications.

Keywords: exosome, exosome-derived miRNA, opthalmic disease, gene diagnosis, gene therapy

1. Introduction

Extracellular vesicles (EVs) are diameter of 30–200 nm sized vesicles secreted by most human cells, and they participate in cell-cell communication, such as antigen presentation, inflammatory factors transmission and tumor proliferation [1]. There are three subtypes of EVs based on size, content and production pathways: Ectosomes (with a diameter of 100 to 1000 nm) are formed by direct plasma membrane budding. Other small extracellular vesicles (sEVs) with a diameter of less than 200 nm are called exosomes. The last subgroup of EVs, ranging from 500 to 5000 nm, are called apoptotic bodies and originate from plasma membrane [2]. In the present review, we mainly discuss the functions and cargoes of exosomes, especially exosome-derived miRNAs, and their relationship with common ophthalmic diseases, and we also discuss standardized methods for EV isolation and potential gene therapy methods for clinical treatments in the future.

1.1 Exosome

Exosome originates from endosomal limiting membranes to form intraluminal vesicles (ILVs), then transport to multivesicular bodies (MVBs) and fused with plasma membrane, finally released as exosomes (see **Figure 1**). Exosomes are secreted by most cell types and have been found in all body fluid such as plasma, urine, semen,

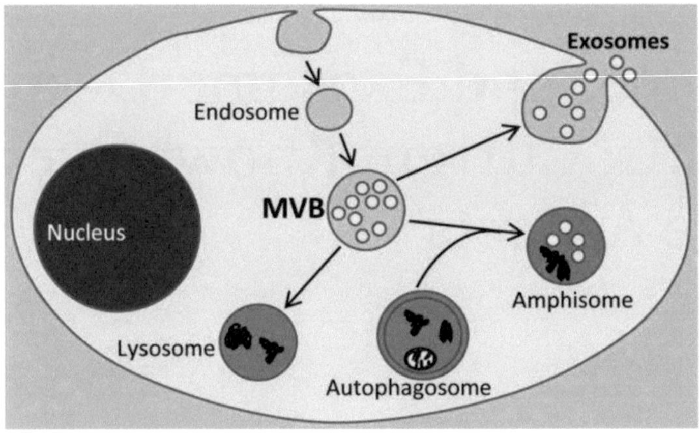

Figure 1.
Exosome release procedure. MVBs, also called late endosomes, fuse with lysosomes, leading toautophagosomes to form amphistomesand then fuse with the plasma membrane. After fusion of MVBs with the plasma membrane the ILVs of MVBs are released as EVs and then called exosomes [3].

saliva, breast milk and tears [4]. Formation and secretion of exosome is regulated through endosomal sorting complexes required for transport (ESCRT) pathway, while the exact mechanism is still remains unclear.

1.2 Composition

Exosomes contain multiple cargoes, including proteins, nucleic acids, lipids. Researchers have identified 9769 proteins, 3408 mRNAs, 2838 miRNAs and 1116 lipids in exosomes [5]. Since the formation and transportation of exosomes are regulated by ESCRT proteins (Alix, TSG101, HSC70 and HSP90β), the above are supposed to marker proteins [6]. Another ESCRT-independent mechanism also releases exosomes into extracellular space via sphingomyelinase enzyme [7]. The CD63, CD9 and CD81 are tetraspanin family proteins and also enriched in exosomes. Others include glycoproteins, posttranslational modifications (PTMs) proteins, Golgi apparatus-associated proteins and endoplasmic reticulum proteins [8].

Several studies have indicated cholesteryl ester (CE), triacylglycerol (TAG) and cardiolipin in exosome contents. The lipid composition and enrichment factors from different cell types are summarized in **Figure 2** by Tore Skotland et al. [3].

1.3 Exosome-derived miRNAs

Exosomes conclude mRNA, noncoding RNA species and DNA. It modulates extracellular environment in physiological or inflammatory state by selectively incorporating specific proteins, mRNA or miRNA to nearby or distant target cells [9]. MiRNAs are a group of single-stranded, 21–25 nucleotide-sized noncoding RNA molecules [10]. MiRNAs are transcribed by RNA polymerase II as primary miRNAs, then processed by RNase III enzyme (Drosha and DGCR8) to single hairpins as precursor miRNAs. Next, the pre-miRNAs are transformed to 20–25 nucleotides long with partial complementarity in the cytoplasm by RNase III enzyme Dicer. The double-stranded miRNAs are transported to the AGO protein family and finish the RNA-induced silencing complex (RISC) loading process, finally becoming a mature

Lipid composition of exosomes released by individual cell types

	PC-3 Cells		PC-3 Cells + HG		Oli-neu Cells		HepG2/C3a		B-Lymphocytes		Mast Cells		Dendritic Cells		Reticulocytes		Platelets	Adipocytes
Lipids	%	Factor	%	Factor	%[a]	Factor	%[a]	Factor	%	Factor	%[b]	Factor	%[b,c]	Factor	%	Factor	%	%[a]
CHOL	43.5	2.3	59	1.7	43	2.3	43	1.9	42.1	3.0	15	1.0	NR	NR	47	1.03	42.5	43
SM	16.3	2.4	9.1	2.0	8.2	1.5	9.7	10.8	23.0	2.3[d]	12	2.8	20	2.2	8.4[d]	1.31	12.5	12.5
PC	15.3	0.31	10.8	0.33	26.7	0.67	20	0.67	(20.3)[e]	(0.76)[e]	28	0.66	26	0.6	23.5	1.03	15.9	33
PS	11.7	2.1	6.9	1.2	14.9	3.0	15.6	2.4	(20.3)[e]	(0.76)[e]	(16)[e]	(1.2)[e]	(19)[e]	(1.6)[e]	5.9	0.92	10.5	1.1
PE	5.8	0.55	1.1	0.21	10.9	1.0	7.4	1.2	(14.6)[e]	(0.7)[e]	24	1.08	26	1.13	12.7	0.84	3.1	4.0
PE ethers	3.3	1.2	4.7	0.81					(14.6)[e]	(0.7)[e]							3.2	
DAG	1.5	1.5	1.1	0.92														0.8
PC ethers	0.81	0.40	0.7	0.28													1.4	
PG	0.17	0.17	0.1	0.07													NR	
PA	0.16	1.8	0.1	0.33					(20.3)[e]	(0.76)[e]							NR	
PI	0.13	0.13	0.3	0.16	NR		4.1	0.18	(20.3)[e]	(0.76)[e]	(16)[e]	(1.2)[e]	(19)[e]	(1.6)[e]	2.4	1.1	5.2	2.3
Cer	0.32	1.3	0.7	1.2	NR	3.3	0.63	2.0									0.40	0.2
HexCer	0.76	3.8	2.3	2.1		2.0												0.02
LacCer	0.12	3.0[f]	0.7	1.8		NR												
Lipid analysis	MS		MS		MS	NR	MS/GC		TLC		TLC/GLC		TLC/GLC		TLC		MS	MS
Exosome preparations[g]	SFM + SUC		SFM + SUC		SFM + SUC + SG		uFCS + SUC + IG		uFCS+ SUC+ SG + immunocapture		uFCS + SUC		uFCS + SUC		uFCS + SUC		SUC + IG	SFM + SUC

%, percent of total lipid quantified; Factor, factor of enrichment from cells to exosomes; DAG, diacylglycerol; NR, not reported; LacCer, lactosylceramide; PA, phosphatidic acid; PG, phosphatidylglycerol; SFM, serum free medium; uFCS, ultracentrifuged FCS; SUC, sequential centrifugation; SG, sucrose gradient; IG, iodixanol gradient.

[a]Percent CHOL not reported; CHOL set to 43% to better compare the content of other lipid classes with the other data shown.

[b]Recalculated from their data.

[c]CHOL not reported; the sum for the other lipid classes is 100% (including LysoPC not included in this table).

[d]Sum of SM and the glycosphingolipid, GM3.

[e]Sum for all classes shown in parentheses and having the same numbers.

[f]Enrichments of other lipid classes are shown in Fig. 2.

[g]Exosome preparations: methods used to isolate the exosome preparations.

Figure 2.
Lipid composition of exosomes released by different cells types were summarized from former review [3].

single-stranded miRNA [11]. Generally, the RICS-miRNA complex pairs with targeted mRNA in the 3′-untranslated region (3′-UTR) sequence. Once combined, miRNA acts either as a mRNA transcription/translation blocker or repressor, or as a promotor for mRNA degradation [12]. The expression of exosome-derived miRNAs profile in a particular cell form is modified in different pathological and physiological conditions [13]. MiRNAs influence cell proliferation, differentiation, apoptosis and metabolism. It regulates approximately 60% of all protein coding genes. Numerous miRNAs derived from circulating exosomes have been proved to be correlated to various diseases, such as cancer and heart failure [14, 15]. It also paly pivotal role in ophthalmic diseases and could be a potential tool in clinical diagnosis, prognostic evaluation or therapeutic target.

2. Exosome-derived miRNAs identified in ophthalmic diseases

2.1 Age-related macular degeneration (dry AMD)

Age-related macular degeneration (AMD) is a progressive retinal degenerative disease and the main cause of irreversible vision blur in elderly people. AMD can be classified into early-phase (non-exudative, dry AMD) and advanced-phase (exudative, wet AMD) forms. Dry AMD is featured with retinal pigment epithelium (RPE) layer dysfunction, photoreceptor degeneration, drusen deposits or geographic atrophy (GA). Dry AMD is the most common type and accounts for 90% of AMD cases. It induces malfunction and atrophy of retinal cells and progresses to advanced AMD to cause visual damage [16–19]. Choroidal neovascularization (CNV) is the hallmark of wet AMD and anti-vascular endothelial growth factor (anti-VEGF) intravitreal injection is the main therapy to suppress CNV development. It has been proved that chronic oxidative stress, retinal cells inflammation and metabolic production aggregation induce exosome function variation, as well as exosome-derived miRNAs deregulation.

Multiple dry AMD samples, such as whole blood, serum and aqueous fluid have been studied to verify miRNAs variations: Three serum-derived miRNAs (*miR-19a, miR-126 and miR-410*) were found increased in dry AMD patients than controls and regulate neurodegenerative signal pathway [20]. Another research proved higher expression of 8 miRNAs (*hsa-let-7a-5p*, *hsa-let-7d-5p*, *hsa-miR-23a-3p*, *hsa-miR-301a-3p*, *hsa-miR-361-5p*, *hsa-miR-27b-3p*, *hsa-miR-874-3p* and *hsa-miR-19b-1-5p*) in serum of dry AMD than controls [16]. Wooff et al. [21] demonstrated that exosome inhibitor impeded the translocation of photoreceptor exosome-derived *miR-124-3p* to the inner retina under photo-oxidative damage. Morris et al. [22] proved that exosome-derived *miR-21* from RPE cells was taken up by microglia, then influenced p53 pathway genes through co-culture of RPE and microglia cells, which indicated that microglia affect AMD progression. Cholesterol-related *miR-33* was found increased in the RPE layer of aging mice, and *miR-33*-targeting *ABCA1* gene may be genetically related to dry AMD [23]. Ren et al. [24] found upregulation of *miR-27a-3p*, *miR-29b-3p* and *miR-195-5p* in 72 dry AMD samples compared to 140 controls and proved the whole blood *miR-27a-3p* to be a diagnostic biomarker for AMD. Litwińska et al. [25] found decreased expression of *miR-16-5p*, *miR-17-3p* and *miR-17-5p* and increased expression of *miR-23a-3p*, *miR-126-3p*, *miR-126-5p* and *miR-146a* in peripheral blood nuclear cells of dry AMD patients. Szemraj et al. [26] reported higher expression of *miR-661*, *miR-3121*, *miR-4258*, *miR-889*, *miR-438*, *miR-424-5p*, *miR-301-5p* and *let-7* in blood serum of dry AMD patients. Ulańczyk et al. [27] proved AMD to be correlated to higher levels of *miR-23a-3p*, *miR-126-5p*, *miR-16-5p*, *miR-17-3p*, *miR-17-5p*, *miR-223-3p*, *miR-93* while lower levels of *miR-21-3p* and *miR-155-5p* in blood plasma samples.

2.2 Age-related macular degeneration (wet AMD)

Exosome-derived miRNAs also mediate wAMD pathology. For instance, Romano et al. [28] found increase of *miR-9* and *miR-34a* in the plasma of wAMD patients. Ménard et al. [29] found increase of *miR-146a* and decrease of *miR-106b*, *miR-152* in the plasma and vitreous humor of wAMD cases. Ertekin et al. [30] found increase of 5 genes (*miR-20a-5p*, *miR-106a-5p*, *miR-24-3p*, *miR-17-5p* and *miR-223-3p*), while decrease of 11 genes (*miR-140-3p*, *miR-21-5p*, *miR-25-3p*, *miR-146b-5p*, *miR-192-5p*, *miR-335-5p*, *miR-342-3p, miR-374a-5p*, *miR-410*, *miR-660-5p* and *miR-574-3p)* in serum of wAMD samples. In vitro research, Maria et al. [31] demonstrated H_2O_2 inhibited *miR-205-5p* and downstream *VEGF* gene function in ARPE-19 cells of wet AMD model.

2.3 Diabetic retinopathy (DR)

Exosome-derived miRNAs influence the development of diabetic retinopathy. Gu et al. [32] proved that *miR-202-5p* secreted by RPE cells mediates TGF/Smad pathway to inhibit endothelial-mesenchymal transition process, which is a promotor to proliferative DR. Another research showed that decrease of *miR-1260b* inhibits vascular smooth muscle cells proliferation and *Notch3* expression, thus may contribute to DR treatment [33]. Qian et al. [34] found that Tsp-1$^+$ retinal microglia cell-derived exosomes negatively regulate *miR-27a-5p* expression and angiogenesis, thus inhibiting DR progression. Xi Chen et al. [35] proved that M1 microglia-derived exosomes enhance neovascularization via *miR-155-5p* by using retinal angiogenesis model. Other exosome-derived miRNAs related to DR in vitro and in vivo are listed in **Table 1**.

Diseases	MicroRNA	Up Regulation	Down Regulation	Target Gene	Model (*In vitro*, *In vivo*, Human)
Diabetic retinopathy	miR-29b	√		RAX	*In vivo*
	miR-195	√		SIRT1	In vitro/ In vivo
	miR-19a	√		IL-10	Human (n = 20)/*In vitro*
	miR-1273 g -3p	√		C5AR2	*In vitro*/*In vivo*
	miR-21	√		PPARα	*In vitro*/*In vivo*
	miR-211	√		SIRT1	Human (n = 40)/*In vivo*
	miR-365	√		Timp3	*In vitro*/*In vivo*
	miR-219 -5p	√		LRH-1	*In vitro*
	miR-21	√		TIMP3	Human/*In vivo*
	miR -200c	√		TLR4 TNF-α IL-1β	*in vivo*
	miR-146a		√	IRAK1	*In vivo*/*In vitro*
	miR-184		√	frizzled-7	*In vitro*/*In vivo*
	miR-7		√	IRS-1	*In vitro*/*In vivo*
	miR-126		√	IRS-1	*In vitro*/*In vivo*
	miR-29a		√	AGT	*In vitro*/*In vivo*
	miR-384-3p		√	hexokinase 2 (HK2)	*In vitro*/*In vivo*
	miR-200b		√	VEGFA	Human (n = 255)/*In vivo*
	miR-199a		√	HIF-1α	*In vivo*
	miR-1983		√	PI3K MAPK Wnt	*In vivo*
	miR-106a		√	HIF1α VEGF	*In vitro*/*In vivo*
	miR- 29a/b		√	Forkhead box protein O4	*In vitro*/*In vivo*
	miR-126		√	HO-1	*In vitro*/*In vivo*
	miR-155	√		TGF-β	Human (n = 60)
	miR-93	√		—	Human (n = 57)
	miR- 200b	√		—	Human (n = 59)

Table 1.
Selected microRNAs involved in retinal diseases [36].

2.4 Other fundus diseases

Several aqueous or retinal exosomes-derived miRNAs have been identified as potential targets for other fundus diseases. For example, increase of *miR-582-3p* in aqueous-derived exosomes may affect cholinergic receptor muscarinic 2 and be a risk factor for the progression of myopia [37]. A higher expression of *miR-148a* was detected in retinal detachment (RD) patients, indicating its potential function in EMT (epithelial-mesenchymal transition) of RPE cells [38]. Similarly, *miR-148a* in vitreous fluid was also found correlated to duration and severity of RD [39]. A global miRNA profiling was performed in a retinitis pigmentosa

(RP) model by Loscher et al. [40], *miR-1, miR-133* were decreased and *miR-96, miR-183* increased, meanwhile novel retinal preference for *miR-376a* and *miR-691* was identified. T Metin et al. [41] detected plasma miRNA levels in 13 premature retinopathy (ROP) infants and found increase of *miR-23a* and *miR-200b-3p*, while decrease of *miR-27b-3p* and *miR-214-3p* in ROP patients. Andrea Russo et al. [42] suggested that deregulation of *miR-19b* and *miR-24* might be correlated to macular hole and epiretinal membrane.

2.5 Glaucoma

Former studies have verified a variety of miRNAs deviations in exosome of glaucoma samples. Peng et al. [43] observed decrease of *miR-200a* in retinal samples from glaucomatous mice model. Jayaram et al. [44] identified 17 dysregulated miRNAs in a mouse model of glaucoma, among them *miR-27a, -29b, -497* and *-16* were associated with retinal ganglion cell (RGC) apoptosis. Li et al. [45] proved protective effect of Müller cell gliosis after optic nerve crush injury by inhibiting *miR-21*. Xiaoyuan Ye et al. [46] demonstrated hypoxia-activated retinal astrocytes to secrete exosomes and exosome-derived *miR-329-5p* protects RGC with apoptosis and retinal ischemia-reperfusion injury.

2.6 Ocular tumors

Ocular tumors are rare but vital to vision and life survival. Intraocular tumors consist of two types: primary and secondary tumors. The former begins primarily in the eyeball; the latter is metastasized from other organs, mainly from breast and lung cancers. Common ocular tumors include retinoblastoma (RB) and uveal melanoma (UM). In tumor cells, exosomes mediate angiogenesis and hypoxia accelerates metastasis by inducing exosomes release. Exosome-derived *miR-105* was proved to depress ZO-1, which increases vascular permeability and tumor metastasis [47]. In a study using UM cell lines, Nannan Liu et al. [48] proved *miR-9* mediates UM's metastasis via NF-kB pathway. Achberger et al. [49] found higher expression of *miR-20a, 125b, 146a, 155, 181a* and *223* in plasma of UM patients. Worley et al. [50] found upregulation of *let-7b, miR-143, 199a, 199a*, 193b and 652* in primary UM tissue, which discriminates patients with class 2 from class 1 UM subtype. For exosome-derived miRNAs, Eldh et al. [51] isolated exosomes from liver perfusate of metastatic UM patients. PCR results showed upregulation of *miR-125b* and *– 25,* which have also been previously reported.

Retinoblastoma (RB) is a primary intraocular tumor and common in children. Zhao et al. [52] screened out *miR-494* to be highly expressed in human RB tissues and involved in tumorigenesis. Jo et al. [53] found upregulation of *miR-29c* in SNOUT-RB1 cells and *let-7i* in Y79 cell lines by bioinformatic analysis, which indicated their roles in RB treatment. A total of 33 miRNAs are both dysregulated in RB tumor and serum samples, of which 25 increase and 8 decrease (see **Figure 3**).

2.7 Cataract

A former study identified more than 10 exosome-derived miRNAs from aqueous humor in patients during cataract surgery, among them *miR-486-5p, miR-204* and *miR-184* are abundant [55].

Upregulated miRNA RB Tumor and RB Serum and Targets Identified in RB Tumor Exosomes		Downregulated miRNA RB Tumor and RB Serum and Targets Identified in RB Tumor Exosomes		miRNA Derived from RB Cell Lines Exosomes and Targets Identified in RB Tumor Exosomes	
miRNA	**Target Gene**	**miRNA**	**Target Gene**	**miRNA**	**Target Gene**
hsa-miR-16-1	KIAA1598	hsa-let-7a	TJP3	hsa-miR-148a	CAMSAP1, IKBIP, NUP50, PPP2R2A
hsa-miR-29b-1	LPGAT1	hsa-miR-92a	INTS1		
hsa-miR-34a	PTRHD1	hsa-let-7f-2	ERCC3, UNC13B		
hsa-miR-96	UNC13B				
hsa-miR-143	ADD3, AK2	hsa-miR-217	ARPC2, EIF1	hsa-miR-582	CACNA2D2, MPP1, NEFL, PIN4, VDAC3
hsa-miR-30d	DCK, POLD3	hsa-let-7a-2	CCNB1, GSTM1, TMEM55B		
hsa-miR-16	OS9, TPPP3	hsa-miR-92a-1	FAM120A, MPDZ, TNR, TPPP3	hsa-miR-200a	CTSV, DAG1, GLRX, MTMR2, PRPS1, SLC27A4, UBXN4
hsa-miR-142	CCNB1, FAM49B, SDHB				
hsa-miR-106b	PPP2R2A, UBXN4, WDR36	hsa-miR-216a	GLRX, POLD3, PPP2R2A, DLG5, PPIF, UNC119		
hsa-miR-182	IKBIP, LMAN2, NUP50				
hsa-miR-183	MPP1, SEC61B, SNAP25				
hsa-miR-148b	MPDZ, TRIM2, DKFZp781M17165, LONP1, PPP1R2	hsa-miR-92a-2	CACNA2D2, MPP1, OS9, P4HTM, PAK1, SIN3B	hsa-miR-483	DCK, DKFZp781M17165, GSTM1, HAUS3, MYDGF, PPP2R1B, PTRHD1
hsa-miR-29c	DAG1, NDUFS6, PDCD4, PPIF, NEFL, PRPS1	hsa-let-7i	DNAJC5, ATP8A1, DAG1, PTRHD1, SLC25A13, TTC9C, UQCRFS1	hsa-miR-216b	ABI2, ATP2B2, ATP8A1, CCDC85C, CISD2, CUX1, DNAJC5, FAM120A, ITSN1, LPGAT1, PPP1R2, RQCD1, TNR, TRMT6, TSPAN14, UBXN7, WIPF2
hsa-miR-30b	CACNA2D2, ERCC3, GSTM1, SLC27A4, TMEM55B, MED4, ARPC2				
hsa-miR-494	ABI2, ATP2B2, ATP6V1C1, ATP8A1, CAMSAP1, CCDC85C, CISD2, CTSV, CUX1, DCC, DLG5, DNAJC5, DPF3, EIF1, FAM120A, GLRX, HAUS3, ITSN1, KDM1B, MTMR2, NCAN, PAK1, QSER1, SLC25A13, UBXN7, WDR11, WIPF2, ARPP19, PEA15, PIN4, PPP2R1B, RQCD1, SIN3B, SYNGR1, TNR, TRMT6, TSPAN14, UNC119, UQCRFS1	hsa-miR-9	ADD3, ARPP19, ATP6V1C1, CCDC85C, CISD2, CTSV, CUX1, DCC, DCK, FAM49B, ITSN1, KDM1B, LPGAT1, MED4, NCAN, PDCD4, PEA15, QSER1, RQCD1, TRIM2, UBXN4, WDR11, ABI2, ATP2B2, CAMSAP1, DKFZp781M17165, DPF3, HAUS3, IKBIP, MTMR2, NEFL, PPP1R2, PRPS1, SLC27A4, SNAP25, TSPAN14, UBXN7, WIPF2	hsa-miR-301b	ADD3ARPP19ATP6V1C1CCNB1DCCDLG5DPF3FAM49BNCANPAK1PEA15QSER1SLC25A13SNAP25TMEM55BTRIM2UQCRFS1WDR11

Figure 3.
The list of miRNA reported in RB tumor, RB serum, and RB cell lines and their targets from the proteins identified in the RB tumor exosomes [54].

3. Exosome isolation methods and exosome-derived miRNAs screening

The overall procedures and methods for exosome isolation have been summarized previously (see **Table 2** and **Figure 4**). In general, exosomes are isolated by ultra-centrifugation-associated methods. Other alternative methods include size-based techniques, immunoaffinity capture methods, precipitation and microfluidic methods. While the above methods are unable to exclusively isolate single-type exosome, as the biological samples are often complex and physiochemical properties are similar between different exosomes.

The most common methods for identifying exosomal miRNAs recently are next-generation sequencing technology (NGS), reverse transcription polymerase chain

Isolation Technique	Recovery	Purity	SampleVolume	TimeRequired
Ultracentrifugation	5–25%	Low	100 s of mLs	8 h
Density gradient	Higher than UC	Similar to UC	Up to 1 mL	20 h
Precipitation kits	N/A	Low	>100 uL	Overnight
ExoChip	N/A	N/A	<400 uL	<2 h
Immunoprecipitation	>99% bead recovery	Higher than UC	Up to1 mL	Overnight
ExoSearch chip	42–97%	Higher than UC	20 uL	40 min
Acoustic nanofilter	>80%	High	50 uL	<30 min

Table 2.
Comparison of exosomal isolation techniques based on recovery, purity, required sample volume, and time required for isolation [4].

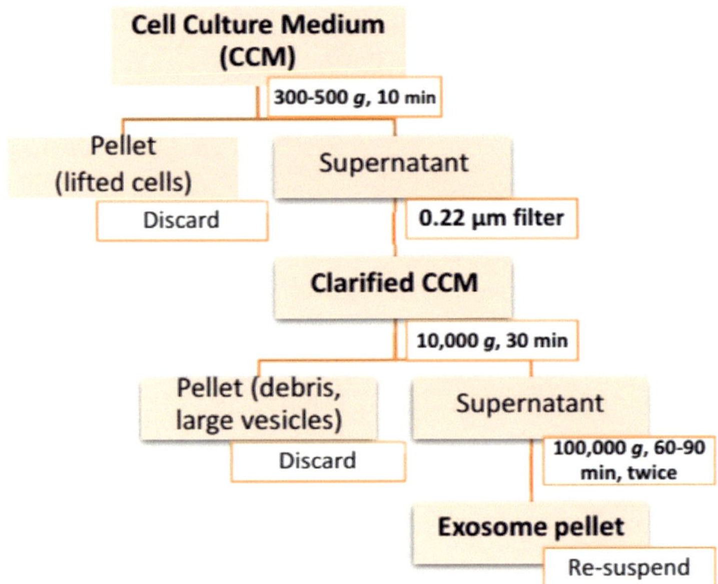

Figure 4.
Workflow of differential ultracentrifugation for exosome isolation [4].

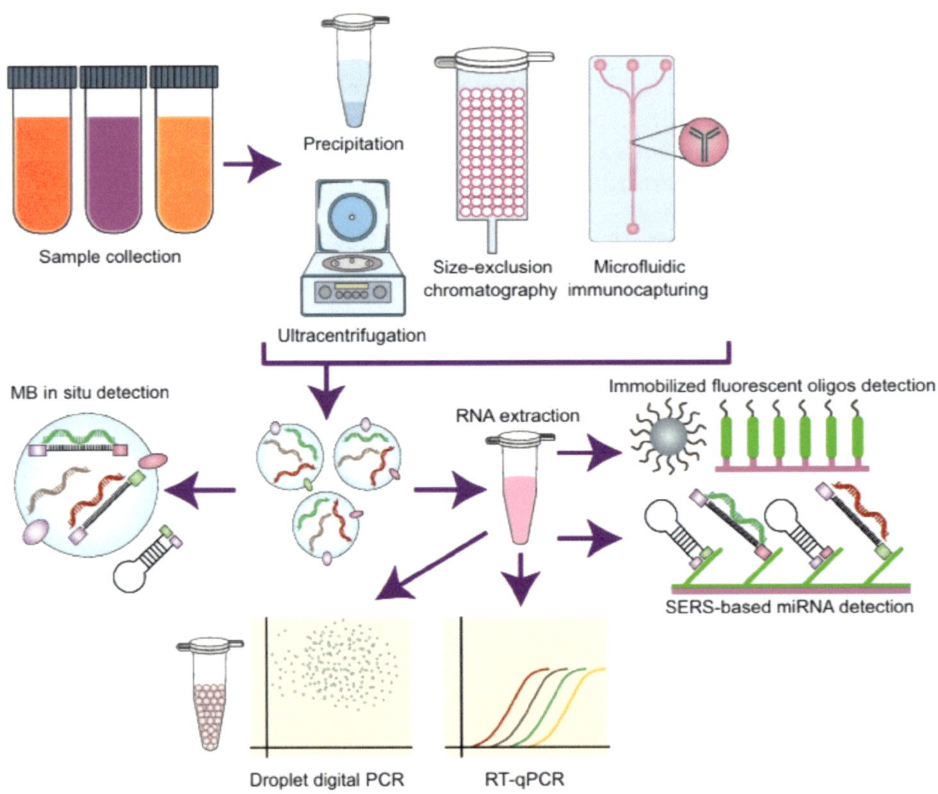

Figure 5.
Overview of methods for characterization and quantification of exosomal miRNAs [56].

reaction (RT-PCR) and digital PCR. But the above methods also have limitations: First, RT-PCR shows low sensitivity and high cost for routine use. Secondly, digital PCR shows high sensitivity but is highly complicated and expensive. Thirdly, NGS requires a complicated pretreatment process. An overview for exosomal miRNAs quantification techniques is shown in (**Figure 5**). Recently, PCR-free approaches have shown promising advantages to conventional methods. For instance, a biotinylated probe on a streptavidin-coated magnetic bead is designed to identify exosomal miRNAs. Another PCR-free approach used molecular beacons (MBs) to quantify miRNAs with fluorescent oligo nucleotides hybridized to targeting miRNA sequence. MBs can also measure miRNAs concentrations in the sample after fixing with a surface-enhanced Raman scattering (SERS) substrate [57]. A newly developed electrochemical miRNAs assay was based on hybridization chain reaction (HCR) with DNA-hairpin probes attached to gold electrode and allows for the detection of minimum levels of target miRNAs.

4. Clinical applications for exosome and exosome-derived miRNAs

4.1 Diagnostic potential

The amount and identity of exosome-derived-miRNAs in healthy and patients are different since miRNAs can be used to diagnose disease in a noninvasive manner. For instance, a familial mutation of *miR-204* is the cause of inherited retinal diseases, such as retinal dystrophy or iris defection [20]. In the above part, we have outlined identified exosomal miRNA variations and their correlation to ophthalmic diseases. A better understanding of miRNA genetics and mutations may help to diagnose disease in a noninvasive way.

4.2 Therapeutic potential

Exosomes and miRNAs are attractive tools for therapeutic development. Exosomes are easily generated, purified and stored. Modified Exosomes are easily derived from cellular source and transmit diverse biomolecular cargos, such as lipids, proteins and nucleic acids or viral vectors. It crosses the blood-retinal barrier without inducing pro-inflammatory response or cardiovascular/cerebrovascular events, thus enabling them to treat fundus diseases effectively [58]. In an acute ischemic optic neuropathies rat model, Mead et al. [59] proved that intravitreally injection of bone marrow stem cells-derived EVs increased RGC survival and axon regeneration, meanwhile reduced axonal loss and dysfunction by delivering miRNAs. Moisseiev et al. [59] found intravitreally injection of mesenchymal stem cells-derived exosomes ameliorated retinal ischemia and neovascularization in an oxygen-induced retinopathy (OIR) model. Engineered exosomes are biocompatible and biostable and deliver purposed cargo to targeted cells in a controllable manner [60]. Mature mRNAs and lncRNAs can also be inserted into exosomes via combination of poly A protein or polycomb repressive complex 2 motifs (EZH1 and EZH2) [20]. Wassmer et al. [61] showed that exosome-adeno-associated virus (Exo-AAV) can be transmitted into the retina of adult mice via intravitreal injection. The Exo-AAV penetrated BRB and delivered AAV to multiple retinal layers, which indicates Exo-AAV may serve as an effective gene delivery carrier in the future.

Since exosomal miRNAs affect various pathological processes, multiple forms of genetic pools have been developed. For instance, subretinal injection of lentiviruses, which deliver anti-angiogenic miRNAs, can suppress CNV formation in vitro. A *miR-204*-encoding AAV was shown to inhibit microglial activation and retinal degeneration in $P347S^{-/-}$ and $AIPL1^{-/-}$ mouse models [62]. Intravitreal injection of *miR-126* mimic and plasmid effectively inhibit *VEGFA mRNA* expression and retinal neovascularization in OIR model. As miRNAs repress target mRNAs and modulate downstream signal pathways, we hypothesize that engineered exosomal miRNAs could show potential advantages in gene therapy and augmentation modality. Interestingly, miRNAs can also induce transdifferentiation of human RPE cells into photoreceptors, indicating an alternative function of reproducing photoreceptors or neural cells by reprogramming RPE cells [63–65]. Future development depends on selecting suitable precursor or mature miRNAs or gene delivery carriers, meanwhile optimizing delivery vectors, such as viral or lipid nanoparticles.

5. Conclusions

In conclusion, exosomes and exosome-derived miRNAs are effective candidates for treating ophthalmic diseases. They monitor pathological environments and regulate physiological activities through a series of mechanisms. Further work is needed to design possible cargo carriers for clinical use.

Acknowledgements

The authors apologize to the investigators and research laboratories whose original studies were not cited because of space limitations.

Conflicts of interest

The authors report no conflicts of interest.

Abbreviations

MVs	microvesicles
MVB	multivesicular bodies
ILVs	intraluminal vesicles
DR	diabetic retinopathy
AMD	age-related macular degeneration
RPE	retinal pigment epithelium
RD	retinal detachment
RGC	retinal ganglion cell

DOI: http://dx.doi.org/10.5772/intechopen.1009102

Author details

Ke Mao
Department of Ophthalmology, Renji Hospital, School of Medicine, Shanghai Jiao Tong University, Shanghai, China

*Address all correspondence to: maoke@renji.com

References

[1] Roccaro AM, Sacco A, Maiso P, Azab AK, Tai YT, Reagan M, et al. BM mesenchymal stromal cell-derived exosomes facilitate multiple myeloma progression. The Journal of Clinical Investigation. 2013;**123**(4):1542-1555

[2] Cully M. Exosome-based candidates move into the clinic. Nature Reviews. Drug Discovery. 2021;**20**(1):6-7

[3] Skotland T, Hessvik NP, Sandvig K, Llorente A. Exosomal lipid composition and the role of ether lipids and phosphoinositides in exosome biology. Journal of Lipid Research. 2019;**60**(1):9-18

[4] Doyle LM, Wang MZ. Overview of extracellular vesicles, their origin, composition, purpose, and methods for exosome isolation and analysis. Cells. 2019;**8**(7):727

[5] Zhou L, Lv T, Zhang Q, Zhu Q, Zhan P, Zhu S, et al. The biology, function and clinical implications of exosomes in lung cancer. Cancer Letters. 2017;**407**:84-92

[6] Morita E, Sandrin V, Chung HY, Morham SG, Gygi SP, Rodesch CK, et al. Human ESCRT and ALIX proteins interact with proteins of the midbody and function in cytokinesis. The EMBO Journal. 2007;**26**(19):4215-4227

[7] Trajkovic K, Hsu C, Chiantia S, Rajendran L, Wenzel D, Wieland F, et al. Ceramide triggers budding of exosome vesicles into multivesicular endosomes. Science. 2008;**319**(5867):1244-1247

[8] Sinha A, Ignatchenko V, Ignatchenko A, Mejia-Guerrero S, Kislinger T. In-depth proteomic analyses of ovarian cancer cell line exosomes reveals differential enrichment of functional categories compared to the NCI 60 proteome. Biochemical and Biophysical Research Communications. 2014;**445**(4):694-701

[9] Abels ER, Breakefield XO. Introduction to extracellular vesicles: Biogenesis, RNA cargo selection, content, release, and uptake. Cellular and Molecular Neurobiology. 2016;**36**(3):301-312

[10] Natoli R, Fernando N. MicroRNA as therapeutics for age-related macular degeneration. Advances in Experimental Medicine and Biology. 2018;**1074**:37-43

[11] Gregory RI, Yan KP, Amuthan G, Chendrimada T, Doratotaj B, Cooch N, et al. The microprocessor complex mediates the genesis of microRNAs. Nature. 2004;**432**(7014):235-240

[12] Li SC, Liao YL, Ho MR, Tsai KW, Lai CH, Lin WC. miRNA arm selection and isomiR distribution in gastric cancer. BMC Genomics. 2012;**13**(Suppl. 1):S13

[13] Du S, Ling H, Guo Z, Cao Q, Song C. Roles of exosomal miRNA in vascular aging. Pharmacological Research. 2021;**165**:105278

[14] Manier S, Liu CJ, Avet-Loiseau H, Park J, Shi J, Campigotto F, et al. Prognostic role of circulating exosomal miRNAs in multiple myeloma. Blood. 2017;**129**(17):2429-2436

[15] Shaihov-Teper O, Ram E, Ballan N, Brzezinski RY, Naftali-Shani N, Masoud R, et al. Extracellular vesicles from epicardial fat facilitate atrial fibrillation. Circulation. 2021;**143**(25):2475-2493

[16] ElShelmani H, Brennan I, Kelly DJ, Keegan D. Differential circulating microRNA expression in age-related macular degeneration. International Journal of Molecular Sciences. 2021a;**22**(22):12321

[17] Tang Y, Kang Y, Zhang X, Cheng C. Mesenchymal stem cell exosomes as nanotherapeutics for dry age-related macular degeneration. Journal of Controlled Release. 2023;**357**:356-370

[18] Tan W, Zou J, Yoshida S, Jiang B, Zhou Y. The role of inflammation in age-related macular degeneration. International Journal of Biological Sciences. 2020;**16**(15):2989-3001

[19] Sarwar S, Clearfield E, Soliman MK, Sadiq MA, Baldwin AJ, Hanout M, et al. Aflibercept for neovascular age-related macular degeneration. Cochrane Database of Systematic Reviews. 2016;**2**(2):CD011346

[20] ElShelmani H, Wride MA, Saad T, Rani S, Kelly DJ, Keegan D. The role of deregulated microRNAs in age-related macular degeneration pathology. Translational Vision Science & Technology. 2021c;**10**(2):12

[21] Wooff Y, Cioanca AV, Chu-Tan JA, Aggio-Bruce R, Schumann U, Natoli R. Small-medium extracellular vesicles and their miRNA cargo in retinal health and degeneration: Mediators of homeostasis, and vehicles for targeted gene therapy. Frontiers in Cellular Neuroscience. 2020;**14**:160

[22] Morris DR, Bounds SE, Liu H, Ding WQ, Chen Y, Liu Y, et al. Exosomal MiRNA transfer between retinal microglia and RPE. International Journal of Molecular Sciences. 2020;**21**(10):3541

[23] Gnanaguru G, Wagschal A, Oh J, Saez-Torres KL, Li T, Temel RE, et al. Targeting of miR-33 ameliorates phenotypes linked to age-related macular degeneration. Molecular Therapy. 2021;**29**(7):2281-2293

[24] Ren C, Liu Q, Wei Q, Cai W, He M, Du Y, et al. Circulating miRNAs as potential biomarkers of age-related macular degeneration. Cellular Physiology and Biochemistry. 2017;**41**(4):1413-1423

[25] Litwińska Z, Sobuś A, Łuczkowska K, Grabowicz A, Mozolewska-Piotrowska K, Safranow K, et al. The interplay between systemic inflammatory factors and microRNAs in age-related macular degeneration. Frontiers in Aging Neuroscience. 2019;**11**:286

[26] Szemraj M, Bielecka-Kowalska A, Oszajca K, Krajewska M, Goś R, Jurowski P, et al. Serum microRNAs as potential biomarkers of AMD. Medical Science Monitor. 2015;**21**:2734-2742

[27] Ulańczyk Z, Sobuś A, Łuczkowska K, Grabowicz A, Mozolewska-Piotrowska K, Safranow K, et al. Associations of microRNAs, angiogenesis-regulating factors and CFH Y402H polymorphism-an attempt to search for systemic biomarkers in age-related macular degeneration. International Journal of Molecular Sciences. 2019;**20**(22):5750

[28] Romano GL, Platania CBM, Drago F, Salomone S, Ragusa M, Barbagallo C, et al. Retinal and circulating miRNAs in age-related macular degeneration: An *in vivo* animal and human study. Frontiers in Pharmacology. 2017;**8**:168

[29] Ménard C, Rezende FA, Miloudi K, Wilson A, Tétreault N, Hardy P, et al. MicroRNA signatures in vitreous humour and plasma of patients

with exudative AMD. Oncotarget. 2016;**7**(15):19171-19184

[30] Ertekin S, Yıldırım O, Dinç E, Ayaz L, Fidancı SB, Tamer L. Evaluation of circulating miRNAs in wet age-related macular degeneration. Molecular Vision. 2014;**20**:1057-1066

[31] Oltra M, Vidal-Gil L, Maisto R, Sancho-Pelluz J, Barcia JM. Oxidative stress-induced angiogenesis is mediated by miR-205-5p. Journal of Cellular and Molecular Medicine. 2020;**24**(2):1428-1436

[32] Gu S, Liu Y, Zou J, Wang W, Wei T, Wang X, et al. Retinal pigment epithelial cells secrete miR-202-5p-containing exosomes to protect against proliferative diabetic retinopathy. Experimental Eye Research. 2020;**201**:108271

[33] Lin X, Li S, Wang YJ, Wang Y, Zhong JY, He JY, et al. Exosomal Notch3 from high glucose-stimulated endothelial cells regulates vascular smooth muscle cells calcification/aging. Life Sciences. 2019;**232**:116582

[34] Luo Q, Jiang Z, Jiang J, Wan L, Li Y, Huang Y, et al. Tsp-1^{+} microglia attenuate retinal neovascularization by maintaining the expression of Smad3 in endothelial cells through exosomes with decreased miR-27a-5p. Theranostics. 2023;**13**(11):3689-3706

[35] Chen X, Wang X, Cui Z, Luo Q, Jiang Z, Huang Y, et al. M1 microglia-derived exosomes promote activation of resting microglia and amplifies proangiogenic effects through Irf1/miR-155-5p/Socs1 axis in the retina. International Journal of Biological Sciences. 2023;**19**(6):1791-1812

[36] Salmaninejad A, Pourali G, Shahini A, Darabi H, Azhdari S. MicroRNA and exosome in retinal-related diseases: Their roles in the pathogenesis and diagnosis. Combinatorial Chemistry & High Throughput Screening. 2022;**25**(2):211-228

[37] Zhang H, Zhang X, Li X. Intraocular exosomes in eye diseases. Current Molecular Medicine. 2022;**22**(6):540-548

[38] Takayama K, Kaneko H, Hwang SJ, Ye F, Higuchi A, Tsunekawa T, et al. Increased ocular levels of MicroRNA-148a in cases of retinal detachment promote epithelial-mesenchymal transition. Investigative Ophthalmology & Visual Science. 2016;**57**(6):2699-2705

[39] Tsunekawa T, Kaneko H, Takayama K, Hwang SJ, Oishi A, Nagasaka Y, et al. Correlation between miR-148 expression in vitreous and severity of rhegmatogenous retinal detachment. BioMed Research International. 2017;**2017**:3427319

[40] Loscher CJ, Hokamp K, Kenna PF, Ivens AC, Humphries P, Palfi A, et al. Altered retinal microRNA expression profile in a mouse model of retinitis pigmentosa. Genome Biology. 2007;**8**(11):R248

[41] Metin T, Dinç E, Görür A, Erdoğan S, Ertekin S, Sarı AA, et al. Evaluation of the plasma microRNA levels in stage 3 premature retinopathy with plus disease: Preliminary study. Eye (London, England). 2018;**32**(2):415-420

[42] Russo A, Ragusa M, Barbagallo C, Longo A, Avitabile T, Uva MG, et al. miRNAs in the vitreous humor of patients affected by idiopathic epiretinal membrane and macular hole. PLoS One. 2017;**12**(3):e0174297

[43] Peng H, Sun YB, Hao JL, Lu CW, Bi MC, Song E. Neuroprotective effects of overexpressed microRNA-200a on

activation of glaucoma-related retinal glial cells and apoptosis of ganglion cells via downregulating FGF7-mediated MAPK signaling pathway. Cellular Signalling. 2019;**54**:179-190

[44] Jayaram H, Cepurna WO, Johnson EC, Morrison JC. microRNA expression in the glaucomatous retina. Investigative Ophthalmology & Visual Science. 2015;**56**(13):7971-7982

[45] Li HJ, Sun ZL, Pan YB, Sun YY, Xu MH, Feng DF. Inhibition of miRNA-21 promotes retinal ganglion cell survival and visual function by modulating Müller cell gliosis after optic nerve crush. Experimental Cell Research. 2019;**375**(2):10-19

[46] Ye X, Liu Y, Chen C, Sun Y, Li F, Fu Y, et al. A novel function and mechanism of ischemia-induced retinal astrocyte-derived exosomes for RGC apoptosis of ischemic retinopathy. Molecular Therapy - Nucleic Acids. 2024;**35**(2):102209

[47] Klingeborn M, Dismuke WM, Bowes Rickman C, Stamer WD. Roles of exosomes in the normal and diseased eye. Progress in Retinal and Eye Research. 2017;**59**:158-177

[48] Liu N, Sun Q, Chen J, Li J, Zeng Y, Zhai S, et al. MicroRNA-9 suppresses uveal melanoma cell migration and invasion through the NF-κB1 pathway. Oncology Reports. 2012;**28**(3):961-968

[49] Achberger S, Aldrich W, Tubbs R, Crabb JW, Singh AD, Triozzi PL. Circulating immune cell and microRNA in patients with uveal melanoma developing metastatic disease. Molecular Immunology. 2014;**58**(2):182-186

[50] Worley LA, Long MD, Onken MD, Harbour JW. micro-RNAs associated with metastasis in uveal melanoma identified by multiplexed microarray profiling. Melanoma Research. 2008;**18**(3):184-190

[51] Beasley AB, Chen FK, Isaacs TW, Gray ES. Future perspectives of uveal melanoma blood based biomarkers. British Journal of Cancer. 2022;**126**(11):1511-1528

[52] Zhao JJ, Yang J, Lin J, Yao N, Zhu Y, Zheng J, et al. Identification of miRNAs associated with tumorigenesis of retinoblastoma by miRNA microarray analysis. Child's Nervous System. 2009;**25**(1):13-20

[53] Jo DH, Kim JH, Park WY, Kim KW, Yu YS, Kim JH. Differential profiles of microRNAs in retinoblastoma cell lines of different proliferation and adherence patterns. Journal of Pediatric Hematology/Oncology. 2011;**33**(7):529-533

[54] Lande K, Gupta J, Ranjan R, Kiran M, Torres Solis LF, Solís Herrera A, et al. Exosomes: Insights from retinoblastoma and other eye cancers. International Journal of Molecular Sciences. 2020;**21**(19):7055

[55] Dismuke WM, Challa P, Navarro I, Stamer WD, Liu Y. Human aqueous humor exosomes. Experimental Eye Research. 2015;**132**:73-77

[56] Rahimian N, Nahand JS, Hamblin MR, Mirzaei H. Exosomal microRNA profiling. Methods in Molecular Biology. 2023;**2595**:13-47

[57] Takimoto T, Taylor GL, Connaris HC, Crennell SJ, Portner A. Role of the hemagglutinin-neuraminidase protein in the mechanism of paramyxovirus-cell membrane fusion. Journal of Virology. 2002;**76**(24):13028-13033

[58] van der Merwe Y, Steketee MB. Extracellular vesicles: Biomarkers,

therapeutics, and vehicles in the visual system. Current Ophthalmology Reports. 2017;**5**(4):276-282

[59] Mead B, Tomarev S. Bone marrow-derived mesenchymal stem cells-derived exosomes promote survival of retinal ganglion cells through miRNA-dependent mechanisms. Stem Cells Translational Medicine. 2017;**6**(4):1273-1285

[60] Moisseiev E, Anderson JD, Oltjen S, Goswami M, Zawadzki RJ, Nolta JA, et al. Protective effect of intravitreal administration of exosomes derived from mesenchymal stem cells on retinal ischemia. Current Eye Research. 2017;**42**(10):1358-1367

[61] Riazifar M, Pone EJ, Lötvall J, Zhao W. Stem cell extracellular vesicles: Extended messages of regeneration. Annual Review of Pharmacology and Toxicology. 2017;**57**:125-154

[62] Wassmer SJ, Carvalho LS, György B, Vandenberghe LH, Maguire CA. Exosome-associated AAV2 vector mediates robust gene delivery into the murine retina upon intravitreal injection. Scientific Reports. 2017;**7**:45329

[63] Fan YY, Liu CH, Wu AL, Chen HC, Hsueh YJ, Chen KJ, et al. MicroRNA-126 inhibits pathological retinal neovascularization via suppressing vascular endothelial growth factor expression in a rat model of retinopathy of prematurity. European Journal of Pharmacology. 2021;**900**:174035

[64] Li B, Jiang H, Li H, hang B, Slaughter M, Yan Z, et al. Direct conversion of adult human retinal pigmented epithelium cells to neurons with photoreceptor properties. Experimental Biology and Medicine (Maywood, N.J.). 2021;**246**(2):240-248

[65] Davari M, Soheili ZS, Samiei S, Sharifi Z, Pirmardan ER. Overexpression of miR-183/−96/−182 triggers neuronal cell fate in human retinal pigment epithelial (hRPE) cells in culture. Biochemical and Biophysical Research Communications. 2017;**483**(1):745-751

Chapter 7

Indications and Surgical Treatments for Inherited Retinal Dystrophies

Pamela Ríos and Cristina Irigoyen

Abstract

Inherited retinal dystrophies (IRD, *see Abbreviations*) are a group of genetic disorders characterized by progressive degeneration of the retina, leading to vision loss. These conditions often present with complications such as posterior subcapsular cataracts (PSC), which can significantly impair vision. Additionally, vitreoretinal (VR) complications such as epiretinal membrane (ERM), vitreomacular traction (VMT), and macular hole (MH) are common. Treatment of these complications is surgical. One of the goals of this chapter will be to focus on the prevalence, surgical indications, and pre- and postoperative evaluation in patients with retinal dystrophies and these complications. The growing importance of gene therapy in recent years is also recognized, particularly as a potential tool for enhancing visual function in patients with IRD. Accessing through subretinal space (SRS), the potential area between the neurosensory retina and the retinal pigment epithelium (RPE), allows direct contact of the drug with photoreceptors and RPE, optimizing the concentration of the drug in these cells. We also want to offer in this chapter an insight into the current subretinal injection.

Keywords: inherited retinal dystrophies, posterior subcapsular cataracts, subretinal injection, surgical treatment, vitreoretinal complications

1. Introduction

IRD are a diverse group of hereditary retinal disorders characterized by photoreceptors (rods and cones) degeneration, which progressively impair vision, often culminating in significant visual loss [1]. In this chapter, we will focus on retinitis pigmentosa (RP) (**Figure 1**), since in addition to being the most common retinal dystrophy [2], most series refer to this retinal dystrophy. However, the findings could be extrapolated to other dystrophies. The first symptom in RP's patients is nyctalopia (night blindness), explained by the primary degeneration of rods. As the disease progresses, the death of an increasing number of rods and cones causes the typical concentric loss of peripheral visual field called "tunnel vision". Macular photoreceptors remain normal until the last stages of the disease, which justifies the preservation of central vision in early stages [2].

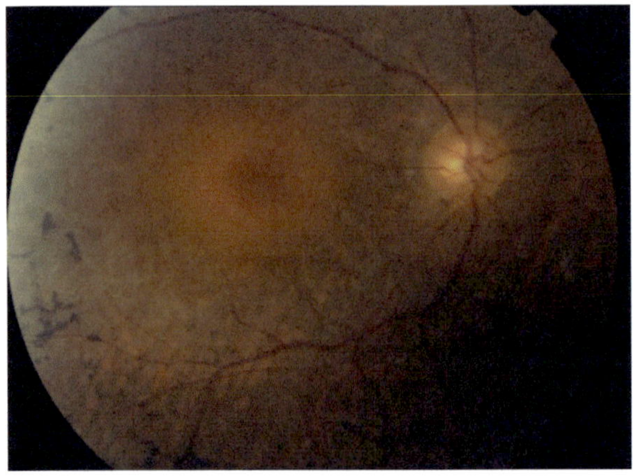

Figure 1.
Retinitis pigmentosa. Fundus with the classic triad: papillary pallor, arteriolar attenuation, and bone-spicule pigment in the mid-peripheral fundus.

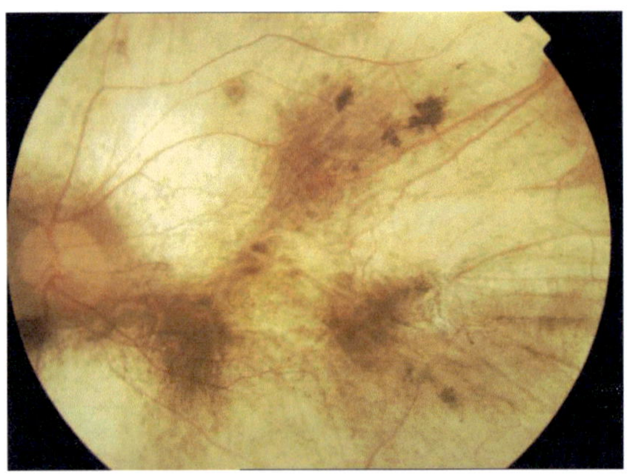

Figure 2.
Choroideremia: Fundus with patchy areas of chorioretinal degeneration in the mid-periphery fundus with preservation of the deep choroidal vessels.

IRD are challenging not only due to their primary retinal manifestations but also because of the secondary complications they have. PSC is one of the most common associated complications in many IRD, including RP (**Figure 1**), Usher syndrome, and choroideremia (**Figure 2**) [3]. Additionally, VR complications such as ERM, VMT, and MH are highly disabling since central vision is often all that is left in RP patients.

The origin and pathophysiological mechanism of PSC formation in RP is unknown. It has been suggested that retinal degeneration produces a hypercellular posterior capsule and the characteristic PSC [4]. The average age at which these patients undergo cataract surgery is earlier: between 47 and 62 years [5].

Most authors agree that cataract surgery helps improve visual acuity (VA) in these patients, which is already impaired due to retinal disease [4–11]. However, various factors have been described that may be responsible for poor visual outcomes after cataract surgery [5, 8, 10, 11]. Therefore, these factors should be analyzed preoperatively to ensure proper surgical indications and to provide patients with realistic expectations regarding postoperative visual results.

The definition of vitreoretinal disorders (VRD) is based on optical coherence tomography (OCT); therefore, its use is essential. ERM is defined as the presence of an epiretinal hyperreflective layer associated to macular contour distortion and/or thickening [12]. VMT an area of vitreous attachment with distortion of the foveal surface [13]. Lamellar macular hole (LMH) is characterized by partial-thickness foveal defect with irregular foveal contour and lamellar separation of the neurosensory retina with cavitation or schisis appearance [14]. VRD were significantly associated with older age, cataract surgery, or presence of cataract [15].

The treatment of VRD is surgical, but the use of dyes, phototoxicity, and potential scar formation has traditionally deterred vitreoretinal surgery in eyes affected by IRD [16]. Nonetheless, given the critical role of pars plana vitrectomy (PPV) in managing VR complications or delivering subretinal drugs, it is important to review ophthalmology literature on this topic.

2. Retinal dystrophies and surgical treatments

2.1 Cataracts In retinal dystrophies

The prevalence of cataracts in RP varies across studies. Fishman et al. demonstrated a 53% prevalence of PSC (including patients who had previously undergone cataract surgery) in a group of 338 patients [17]. Heckenlively et al. found a 41% prevalence of PSC in a group of 291 patients with different IRD; specifically, 31% of patients with choroideremia had cataracts, 42% in the Usher syndrome group, and 28% in the cone and rod dystrophy group [3]. Chatterjee et al. represented the largest cohort of RP patients undergoing cataract surgery in a developing country (India), and differing from the more common PSC reported in other studies, the most prevalent types of cataracts were nuclear sclerosis in 44 (33.3%) eyes. This is attributed to the study's tropical climate and chronic sunlight exposure [18]. In an epidemiological study conducted in Gipuzkoa, Spain, with 164 patients affected by RP, 62% had cataracts or had undergone cataract surgery. No differences were found between sexes in the prevalence of cataracts. There also do not appear to be differences based on mutation type, although the sample size is insufficient.

Fishman et al. demonstrated a probability of 41% (in autosomic dominant (AD)- RP) to 90% (in X-linked (XL) - RP) of having cataracts by age 40, while the likelihood of having cataracts by age 60 reaches over 80% in many genetic types of RP [17]. In our study, 62% of patients had cataracts at the time of the study. However, we observe that if we adjust cataract cases by age groups, this percentage increases significantly with age, with 50–81% of patients expected to have cataracts starting from age 40. In **Figure 3**, we show the prevalence of cataract adjusting for age groups and according to the type of inheritance.

From 0 to 19 years, no patients had cataracts, although there are no patients in the XL- RP group for this age range to assess. Jackson et al., in a retrospective study of 142 eyes, found that the age of cataract surgery was advanced by 10 years in patients with X-linked RP [7].

In conclusion, patients with X-linked RP appear to develop cataracts more frequently and at younger ages compared to other hereditary types of RP and more than 50% of the RP population will develop cataracts by age 40 [3, 17].

The main symptom of PSC is glare, which can further impair the visual function of these patients who already have a visual field altered by the disease [3]. Glare is

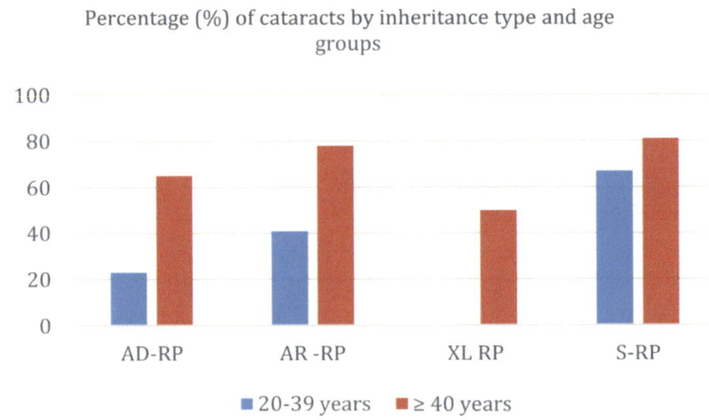

Figure 3.
Prevalence of cataract according to type of inheritance by age group. AR-RP: Autosomal Recessive RP. S-RP: Sporadic retinosis pigmentosa.

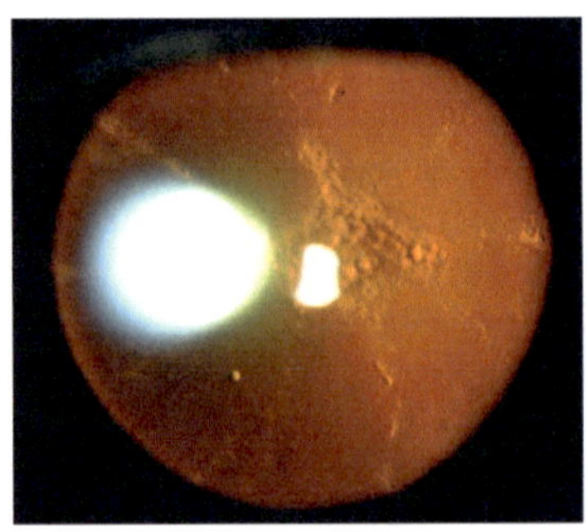

Figure 4.
Posterior subcapsular cataract (PSC): Opacification in the posterior portion of the crystalline lens. It has been suggested that retinal degeneration produces a hypercellular posterior capsule and the characteristic PSC.

accentuated in bright conditions because the PSC becomes more evident with the pupil in miosis. Near vision is more affected than distant vision, and some patients may experience monocular diplopia. The diagnosis of cataracts is clinical, based on the observation of posterior capsule opacification using a slit lamp, as shown in **Figure 4**.

2.2 Preoperative evaluation and predictive factors of visual outcomes in cataract surgery

Most patients benefit from cataract surgery, but evaluating the visual potential in patients with RP can be difficult. In a retrospective study, Bastek et al. demonstrated an improvement in VA of at least 2 lines on the Snellen scale in 83% of the patients who underwent surgery; 52% of the eyes achieved a VA of 20/50 or better. Postoperative visual fields did not change [6]. However, it has also been reported that VA did not improve in 12.5% to 53.6% of eyes in different studies [5, 7]. Although in these studies, after interviewing patients, a subjective improvement was observed in 83–96% of patients [5, 6]. Therefore, other measures of visual function are necessary to evaluate the benefit of cataract surgery in these patients.

Different factors have been described that can worsen vision after cataract surgery:

1. Posterior capsule opacification [5].

2. Anterior capsule contraction as shown in **Figure 5** [19].

3. Zonular weakness and intraocular lens (IOL) dislocation as shown in **Figure 5** [8, 20]

4. Outer retinal atrophy in advanced RP [5]

5. Cystoid macular edema (CEM) in 10–15% [7, 15]

6. Phototoxic retinal damage during surgery [21].

Therefore, a proper preoperative evaluation is important, and the patient should be warned and informed about the potential risks of the surgery and the uncertain prognosis of the visual outcome, primarily depending on the macular condition. The informed consent should provide information about the uncertain prognosis regarding the improvement of VA. In **Table 1**, we summarize the preoperative evaluation of a patient with RP who is going to undergo cataract surgery.

Considering these potential preoperative tests, Yoshida et al. [5] have recently published some possible predictive factors for evaluating the postoperative visual outcome. After analyzing 56 eyes with RP preoperatively using Spectral Domain (SD) OCT and perimetry, they found that the preoperative MD value in the Humphrey Field Analyzer 10–2 program and final VA were significantly correlated, and VA improved significantly in the group with less advanced RP (MD $\geq$ [-15 dB]) as shown in **Figure 6**. The final VA was significantly better in the group where preoperative SD-OCT showed a normal EZ (Grade 3) compared to the groups with a discontinuous ellipsoid zone (Grade 2) or no visible zone (Grade 1). This latter finding was also demonstrated by other authors [10], and they associated EZ integrity with good visual recovery after surgery and observed a correlation between the length of EZ and postoperative VA (the greater the length, the better the postoperative VA) and between central foveal thickness (the greater the thickness, the better the postoperative VA). In this study, patients with macular edema and ERM, which can alter the measurement of central foveal thickness, were excluded.

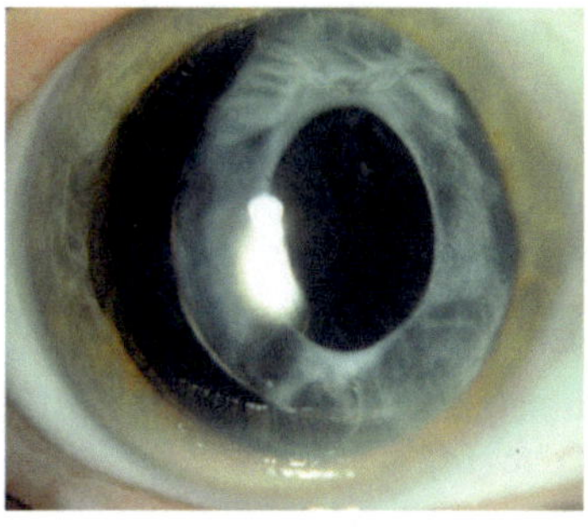

Figure 5.
Subluxated IOL, with anterior capsule contraction and posterior capsulotomy in a patient with RP.

Anamnesis	Eye examination and tests:
Date of central VA decrease [6]: If the patient reports severe VA reduction (requiring low vision aids) in childhood or early adulthood, it is likely that the patient will not recover VA after surgery.	**VA after pupil dilation**: If there is an improvement in VA after pupil dilation, it may indicate PSC [3]. Detect **signs of phacodonesis** to minimize stress on the zonular fibers during cataract surgery [8, 22]
Rate of progression of VA decrease: RP is a slowly progressive disease, so if rapid vision loss is documented after 40, it may indicate cataract development.	**OCT:** Presence of CME and ERM (common in patients with RP) [5] and classification of the ellipsoid zone (EZ) [23]: • Grade 1: Ellipsoid zone not visible • Grade 2: Ellipsoid zone abnormal or discontinuous • Grade 3: Normal ellipsoid zone.
Symptoms: Glare and progressive myopization.	**Autofluorescence (AF)**: Vision and retinal sensitivity reduction have been correlated with the reduction of the area and diameter of the AF ring observed in some RP patients [24].
	Humphrey perimetry: The mean deviation (MD) value in the central 10–2 program analyzes the sensitivity distribution in the macular area to monitor RP progression. Patients with RP and MD values of −15 dB or higher tend to have better VA [25].

Table 1.
Preoperative evaluation in a patient with RP and cataract: Factors to consider for visual prognosis after cataract surgery.

2.3 Vitreoretinal complications in retinal dystrophies

Most studies agree on the prevalence of VRD in RP patients. Fragiotta et al. studied a total of 257 eyes of 145 RP patients, finding 18.3% of cases with VR disorders, including ERM, VMT, and MH [12]. The most common is ERM: studies have found prevalence of 15–20% [15, 26, 27]. The prevalence of VRD is similar to non-tractional CME (20,4%) [15]. Since it is not susceptible to surgical treatment, we will not discuss this complication in this chapter. VR disorders are more prevalent in RP eyes compared to the general population [15], so it is important to assess OCT in patients with RP, especially when central vision have been affected. The pathogenetic process that leads to an increased prevalence of VRD in IRD is still not completely understood.

Patients with IRD and VR complications can be asymptomatic or experience symptoms ranging from mild floaters to metamorphopsia and consequent central vision loss, depending on the degree and depth of retinal disorder. The diagnosis of VR disorders is made through OCT. ERM is defined as a hyperreflective membrane formed by myofibroblast-like cells and collagen fibrils, covering the inner limiting membrane (ILM), and causing distortion of the normal retinal structure [28], as shown in the **Figures** 7 and **8**.

Lamellar macular hole (LMH) is defined by a foveal defect that affects only part of the retinal thickness, resulting in an irregular foveal shape and lamellar separation of the neurosensory retina. This separation can present either a schisis-like or cavitated appearance. In the schisis-like form, hyperreflective bridges span across hyporreflective space, whereas the cavitated form is characterized by a uniformly hyporreflective space within the neurosensory retina [12]. LMH can be associated with an ERM (as previously mentioned, a thin, hyperreflective line over the ILM). However, there is

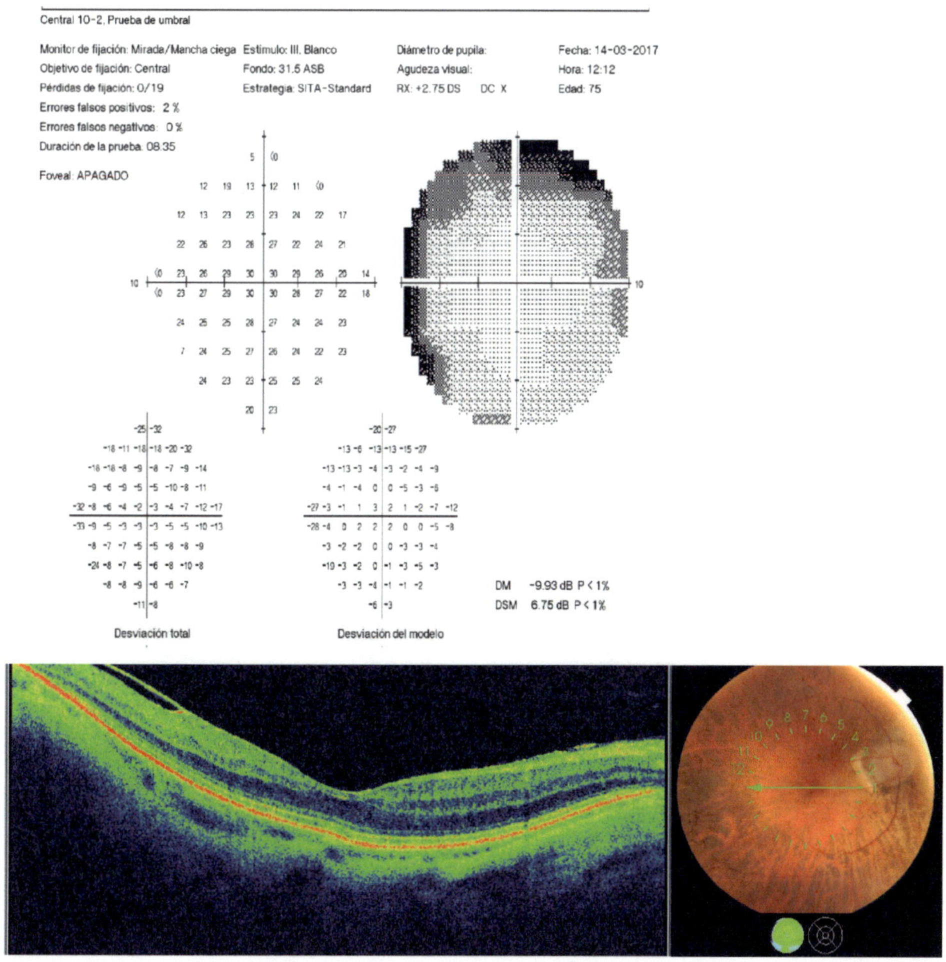

Figure 6.
Patient with RP, showing MD greater than −15 dB in the central visual field (Humphrey 10–2) and preservation of EZ (Grade 3) in the SD-OCT, who, after cataract surgery, recovered VA from 20/50 to 20/25 on the Snellen scale.

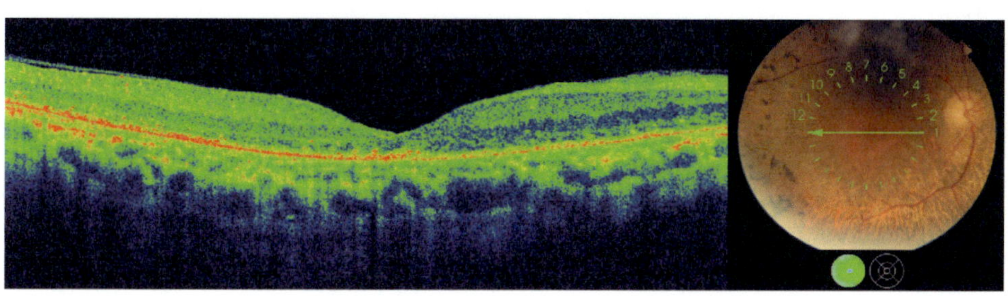

Figure 7.
Patient with a VA of 20/200 on the Snellen scale, who after cataract surgery improved to 20/70. SD-OCT shows a non-visible EZ (Grade 1).

a condition known as lamellar hole associated with epiretinal proliferation (LHEP) shown in **Figure 9**, in which this proliferation is observed between nerve fiber layer and epiretinal surface, appearing as a medium reflectivity material, measuring at

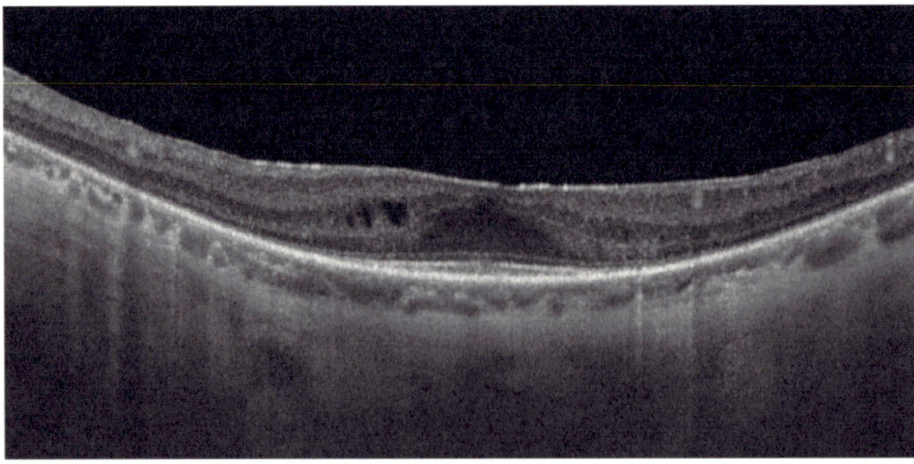

Figure 8.
SD-OCT of a patient with RP and ERM: We can observe the thin hyperreflective (white) line over the ILM, which leads to a disruption of the retinal structure. It is also possible to observe some intraretinal cysts.

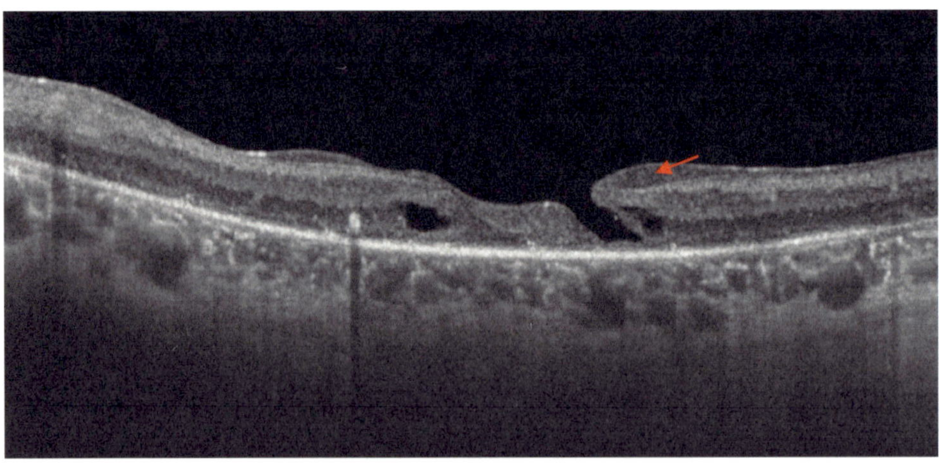

Figure 9.
SD-OCT of a patient with RP and LHEP: A lamellar hole is observed as a partial-thickness foveal defect with an irregular foveal contour, and epiretinal proliferation as a medium reflectivity material (red arrow).

least 20 μm (thicker than ERM) [29, 30]. A full-thickness defect in the central macula is referred to as an MH and is characterized by the disruption of both the inner and outer retinal layers. In patients with RP, MH is primarily caused by CME, incomplete vitreous detachment, and traction from condensed vitreous strands [31, 32].

VMT is defined as an area of vitreous attachment with distortion of the foveal surface and may or may not be associated with an ERM. Adhesion was further divided into focal if 1500 μm or less; or broad, if more than 1500 μm [13]. This classification is important as it helps guide the management of VMT: Focal VMT typically causes localized distortion, leading to changes such as pseudocyst formation and foveal elevation, as shown in **Figure 10**. It often results in fewer visual symptoms and tends to resolve spontaneously, whereas broad VMT can result in more significant anatomical changes and potentially lead to macular edema or MH, both of which can severely affect vision [33].

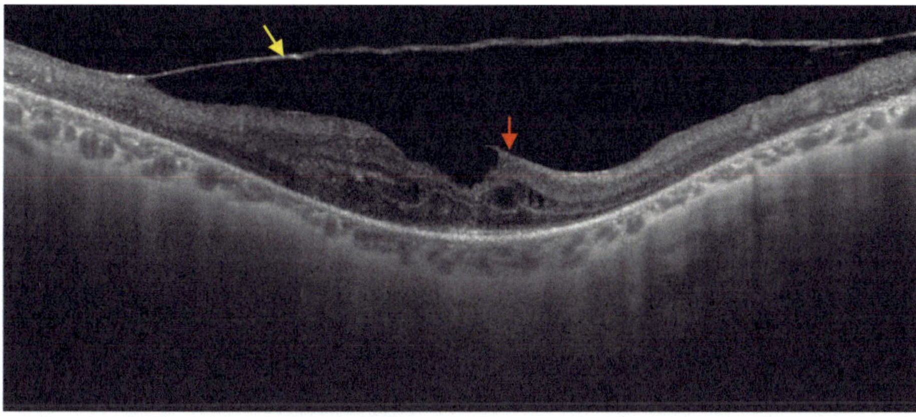

Figure 10.
SD-OCT of a RP patient: VMT associated to a ERM (yellow arrow) with free fovea (red arrow) is observed. Foveal traction likely occurred previously, as foveal distortion and pseudocyst formation are observed. Monitoring these cases with regular OCT and follow-ups is important.

Fragiotta et al. studied VRD and their progression over time, concluding that over a 24-month follow-up, 30–40% of patients with VRD lost one or more lines of best-corrected visual acuity. The ERM subgroup experienced the most significant visual decline, with 39.1% losing one to three lines of vision (VMT: 28.6% lost one line, LM: 8.6% lost three lines) [12]. This directly impacts the quality of life of RP patients, as macular pathology results in central vision loss, compounding the peripheral vision loss already caused by the retinal disease.

Normally, anomalous posterior vitreous detachment (PVD) is considered a key factor in the development of VRD [34]. However, it has been observed a lower prevalence of PVD in patient with RP and VRD (18%) [12]. This suggests that factors such as inflammation, rather than just mechanical issues like PVD, may play a significant role in the high prevalence of VRD in these patients.

2.4 Vitroretinal surgery: Indications, visual outcomes, and toxicity

The decision to perform PPV in patients with IRD is challenging. Surgical indications may be based on the presence of metamorphopsia and decreased visual acuity. However, it is often unclear whether these symptoms are due to VR alterations, cataracts (if patient has not undergone phacoemulsification (PE) yet), or retinal dystrophy itself. A crucial factor to consider during preoperative evaluation is the integrity of EZ, as its condition significantly influences postoperative visual outcomes [35]. The EZ is a hyperreflective line located below the outer nuclear layer and above RPE and reflects the integrity of the photoreceptors. It is common for patients with RPE to have macular disruption of EZ, while preserving subfoveal EZ, during early stages of the disease, as shown in **Figure 11**. As the disease progresses, there is greater photoreceptor involvement, leading to complete disruption of the EZ as shown in **Figure 12**. Other authors suggest postoperative visual and functional outcomes are variable and unpredictable and that EZ is not a reliable predictor of visual outcomes. They concluded regardless of whether the postoperative visual outcomes remain unchanged, decreased, or improved, in most cases, EZ grades did not change. This suggests that other factors, beyond the EZ, may influence outcomes and have not yet

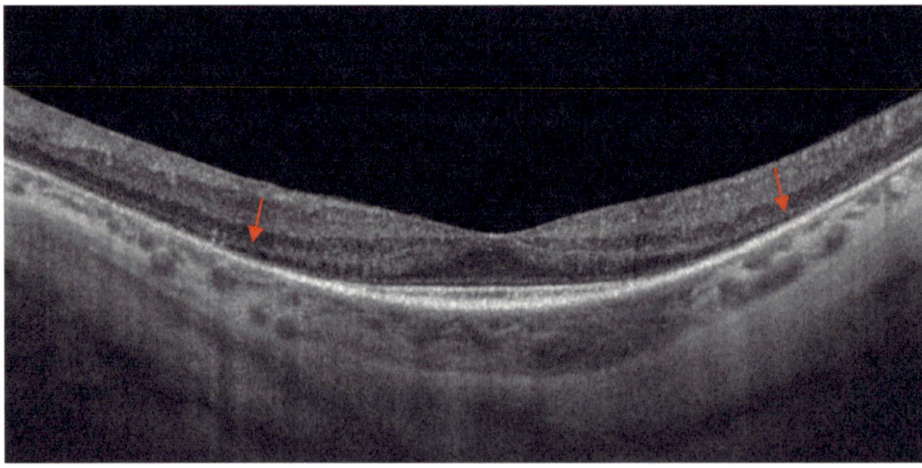

Figure 11.
SD-OCT of patient affected with RP: Disruption of EZ in parafoveal area (red arrow), while preserving integrity of EZ in subfoveal area. Patient has good central vision with AV of 20/50 on the Snellen scale.

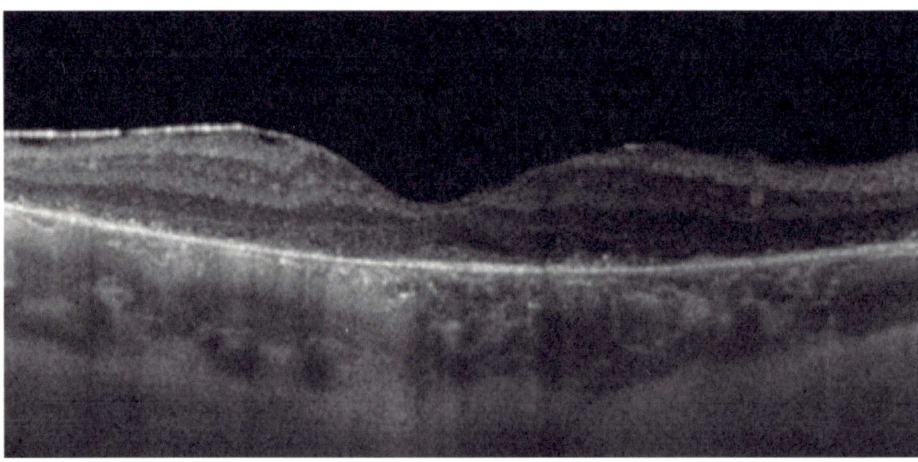

Figure 12.
SD-OCT of a patient with advanced RP: Disruption of EZ in subfoveal and parafoveal area. Probably, this patient would not be a candidate for VR surgery, given the poor visual prognosis, due to significant photoreceptor loss.

been fully studied [36]. Further research is needed to identify these additional factors that may affect visual recovery in these patients.

There is limited evidence regarding VR surgeries and visual outcomes in patients with RD. The results are summarized in **Table 2**.

In most studies, VR surgery has been combined with PE, making it difficult to determine how much of the visual improvement is attributable to VR surgery versus PE. In our experience, and in agreement with other authors [31, 36, 37], a key factor in deciding surgical treatment on ERM is when it is associated with VMT and/or cataracts, which improves visual outcomes. Some authors advocate for combined surgery, suggesting photoreceptor preservation due to diffusible substances or growth factors originating from the stimulated iris, ciliary body, and the retina [41, 42]. In contrast, studies with fewer PE cases showed poorer visual outcomes [35].

Study	Number of eyes and diagnosis	Combined surgery (PPV + PE)	Visual Outcomes
ERM			
Vingolo et al. [37]	8 ERM + VMT	Yes (5/8)	Improved (8/8)
Ikeda et al. [35]	11 ERM	Yes (5/11)	Unchanged (6/11; 3 of these with combined surgery)
Yan et al. [36]	7 ERM + VMT	Yes (7/7)	Improved (6/7)
MH			
Vingolo et al. [31]	3 VMT + MH	Yes (3/3)	Improved (3/3)
Hagiwara et al. [26]	2 MH	Yes (2/2)	Improved (1/2)
Jin et al. [38]	3 MH	No (0/3)	Improved (3/3)
Yan et al. [36]	4 VMT + MH	Yes (4/4)	Improved (2/4)
García-Fernandez et al. [39]	1 MH	No (0/1)	Unchanged
Lee et al. [40]	2 MH	Yes (2/2)	Improved (2/2)

Table 2.
Surgical management of vitreoretinal complications and visual outcomes.

Regarding the surgical technique, most studies performed PPV + ILM peeling, whether for ERM extraction or MH closure. Flap-assisted techniques for RP with MH have shown favorable visual outcomes [40], but larger sample sizes are needed to validate this promising technique. Additionally, the use of dyes, light toxicity, and the risk of retinal atrophy has historically discouraged VR surgery in IRD eyes [16]. However, given the importance of PPV, especially for treating VRD and delivering subretinal drugs, it is important to find solutions for these problems. Phototoxicity has been reduced with modern techniques like xenon light sources and light emitting diodes (LED) lighting with spectral filters [43]. Safer dye alternatives such as Brilliant Blue G (BBG) instead of Indocyanine Green (ICG) show reduced retinal degeneration [35, 36, 43, 44]. Also, ILM peeling without dyes is also recommended to prevent chromotoxicity, but visual outcomes may not be as favorable [37].

2.5 Gene therapy and subretinal injection via vitrectomy

Currently, 280 genes have been associated with IRD, whose mutations impair the function of photoreceptors and RPE [45]. These genetic alterations impair essential retinal processes, making them prime targets for therapeutic intervention. Gene therapy presents a promising approach by modifying gene expression, typically using viral vectors. Adeno-associated virus (AAV), a small, nonpathogenic dependovirus, has emerged as the preferred vector for delivering gene therapies to SRS, due to its favorable safety profile [46].

In 2017, a phase III clinical trial marked a milestone by demonstrating that subretinal injection of a gene therapy called voretigene neparvovec (VN) mediated by AAV2, improved visual function in patients with biallelic mutations in the RPE65 gene. *Luxturna* (the trade name of VN) became the first ocular gene therapy to reach the market [47, 48].

The SRS, located between the neurosensory retina and the RPE, offers a strategic site for drug delivery by ensuring direct access to both photoreceptor and RPE layers, thereby enhancing drug concentration within these target cells. Compared to the intravitreal space, the SRS presents fewer risks due to its enclosed anatomical structure and immune-privileged environment. Additionally, this route requires lower therapeutic doses, making it more efficient for targeted treatments [49]. We want to offer in this chapter an insight into surgical technique of subretinal injection of *Luxterna via* vitrectomy [45, 50–55]. We aim to summarize the steps in **Figure 13**.

Based on our experience as a reference center for IRD in Spain and consistent with other authors [51, 52, 56, 57], we believe there are several key points to consider when performing subretinal injection technique:

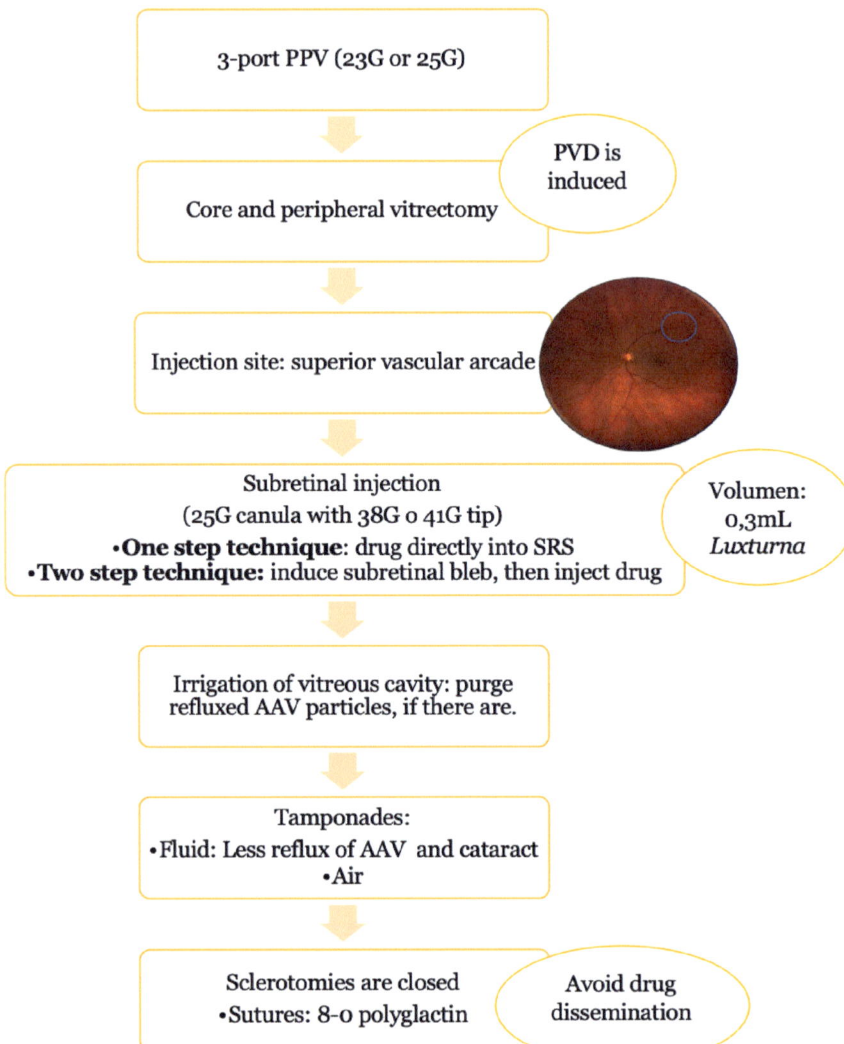

Figure 13.
Steps of Luxturna subretinal injection technique: We preferred one-step technique. Complications of two-steps are enlargement of the initial retinotomy (leading to unintended diffusion of the drug), creation of a second retinotomy, and retinal overstretching, which carries the risk of a macular hole [51].

- Preoperative OCT is essential to avoid injections in areas of retinal atrophy, where the risk of retinal detachment is higher and because it is pointless to administer the drug in regions where photoreceptors are already dead.

- Air bubbles in the cannula must always be purged (ensure this is verified before inserting the instruments into the eye).

- We reserve two-step technique specifically for choroideremia cases, due the enlarge atrophy.

- Intraoperative OCT is a valuable tool that, if available, should be used. It helps determine the needle's depth within the retina, ensuring the injection is precisely within the subretinal space.

- Following the iatrogenic retinal detachment induced during subretinal injections, the subretinal fluid is typically reabsorbed within one day, and the retina restores both its morphology and function within 3–4 weeks.

It is important to highlight that subretinal injection induces an iatrogenic retinal detachment. However, when performed carefully and by experts, the procedure causes minimal trauma and supports rapid recovery of the retina, indicating that it is generally a safe technique [58].

3. Conclusions

- PSC are one of the most common complications in IRD, affecting over 50% of patients with RP by the age of 40.

- Most patients benefit from cataract surgery, though they should be informed of potential complications, such as posterior capsular opacification, anterior capsular contraction, IOL dislocation, and macular edema.

- VRD (ERM, VMT, and MH) are more prevalent in RP eyes compared to the general population, so it is important to assess OCT in these patients, especially when central vision have been affected.

- VR surgery decisions are challenging, particularly with the limited evidence and variable visual outcomes.

- Nowadays, with the ongoing evolving field of gene therapy, it is essential to understand subretinal injection techniques *via* vitrectomy for delivering drugs.

Conflict of interest

The authors declare no conflict of interest.

Abbreviations

AAV	adeno-associated virus
AD	autosomic dominant
AF	autofluorescence
BBG	brilliant blue G
CME	cystoid macular edema
ERM	epiretinal membrane
EZ	ellipsoid zone
ICG	indocyanine green
IRD	inherited retinal dystrophies
ILM	inner limiting membrane
IOL	intraocular lens
LED	light emitting diodes
LHEP	lamellar hole epiretinal proliferation
LMH	lamellar macular hole
MD	mean deviation
MH	macular hole
OCT	optical coherence tomography
PE	phacoemulsification
PPV	pars plana vitrectomy
PSC	posterior subcapsular cataracts
RP	retinitis pigmentosa
RPE	retinal pigment epithelium
SD	spectral domain
SRS	subretinal space
VA	visual acuity
VMT	vitreomacular traction
VN	voretigene neparvovec
VR	vitreoretinal
VRD	vitreoretinal disorders
XL	X-linked

Author details

Pamela Ríos[1*] and Cristina Irigoyen[1,2,3]

1 Department of Ophthalmology, Donostia University Hospital, Donostia-San Sebastián, Spain

2 Biodonostia Health Research Institute, Donostia-San Sebastián, Spain

3 Department of Ophthalmology, University of the Basque Country, Leioa, Spain

*Address all correspondence to: pamelafrancisca.riosfriz@osakidetza.eus

References

[1] Vingolo EM, Mascolo S, Miccichè F, Manco G. Retinitis pigmentosa: From pathomolecular mechanisms to therapeutic strategies. Medicina (Kaunas, Lithuania). 2024;**60**(1):189. DOI: 10.3390/medicina60010189

[2] Dias MF, Joo K, Kemp JA, Fialho SL, da Silva Cunha A Jr, Woo SJ, et al. Molecular genetics and emerging therapies for retinitis pigmentosa: Basic research and clinical perspectives. Progress in Retinal and Eye Research. 2018;**63**:107-131. DOI: 10.1016/j.preteyeres.2017.10.004. Epub 2017 Oct 31. Erratum in: Prog Retin Eye Res. 2018 Sep;66:220-221. doi: 10.1016/j.preteyeres.2018.08.001

[3] Heckenlively J. The frequency of posterior subcapsular cataract in the hereditary retinal degenerations. American Journal of Ophthalmology. 1982;**93**(6):733-738. DOI: 10.1016/0002-9394(82)90469-x

[4] Fagerholm PP, Philipson BT. Cataract in retinitis pigmentosa. An analysis of cataract surgery results and pathological lens changes. Acta Ophthalmologica. 1985;**63**(1):50-58. DOI: 10.1111/j.1755-3768.1985.tb05215.x

[5] Yoshida N, Ikeda Y, Murakami Y, Nakatake S, Fujiwara K, Notomi S, et al. Factors affecting visual acuity after cataract surgery in patients with retinitis pigmentosa. Ophthalmology. 2015;**122**(5):903-908. DOI: 10.1016/j.ophtha.2014.12.003. Epub 2015 Jan 17

[6] Bastek JV, Heckenlively JR, Straatsma BR. Cataract surgery in retinitis pigmentosa patients. Ophthalmology. 1982;**89**(8):880-884. DOI: 10.1016/s0161-6420(82)34700-4

[7] Jackson H, Garway-Heath D, Rosen P, Bird AC, Tuft SJ. Outcome of cataract surgery in patients with retinitis pigmentosa. The British Journal of Ophthalmology. 2001;**85**(8):936-938. DOI: 10.1136/bjo.85.8.936

[8] Dikopf MS, Chow CC, Mieler WF, Tu EY. Cataract extraction outcomes and the prevalence of zonular insufficiency in retinitis pigmentosa. American Journal of Ophthalmology. 2013;**156**(1):82-88.e2. DOI: 10.1016/j.ajo.2013.02.002. Epub 2013 Apr 28

[9] Edwards TL, Groppe M, MacLaren RE. Outcomes following cataract surgery in choroideremia. Eye (London, England). 2015;**29**(4):460-464. DOI: 10.1038/eye.2014.326. Epub 2015 Jan 16

[10] Nakamura Y, Mitamura Y, Hagiwara A, Kumagai K, Miura G, Sugawara T, et al. Relationship between retinal microstructures and visual acuity after cataract surgery in patients with retinitis pigmentosa. The British Journal of Ophthalmology. 2015;**99**(4):508-511. DOI: 10.1136/bjophthalmol-2013-304819. Epub 2014 Oct 21

[11] Yoshida N, Ikeda Y, Notomi S, Ishikawa K, Murakami Y, Hisatomi T, et al. Clinical evidence of sustained chronic inflammatory reaction in retinitis pigmentosa. Ophthalmology. 2013;**120**(1):100-105. DOI: 10.1016/j.ophtha.2012.07.006. Epub 2012 Sep 15

[12] Fragiotta S, Rossi T, Carnevale C, Cutini A, Tricarico S, Casillo L, et al. Vitreo-macular interface disorders in retinitis pigmentosa. Graefe's Archive for Clinical and Experimental Ophthalmology. 2019;**257**(10):2137-2146. DOI: 10.1007/s00417-019-04418-8. Epub 2019 Jul 19

[13] Duker JS, Kaiser PK, Binder S, de Smet MD, Gaudric A, Reichel E, et al. The international vitreomacular traction study group classification of vitreomacular adhesion, traction, and macular hole. Ophthalmology. 2013;**120**(12):2611-2619. DOI: 10.1016/j.ophtha.2013.07.042. Epub 2013 Sep 17

[14] Bottoni F, Deiro AP, Giani A, Orini C, Cigada M, Staurenghi G. The natural history of lamellar macular holes: A spectral domain optical coherence tomography study. Graefe's Archive for Clinical and Experimental Ophthalmology. 2013;**251**(2):467-475. DOI: 10.1007/s00417-012-2044-2. Epub 2012 May 9

[15] Testa F, Rossi S, Colucci R, Gallo B, Di Iorio V, Della Corte M, et al. Macular abnormalities in Italian patients with retinitis pigmentosa. The British Journal of Ophthalmology. 2014;**98**(7):946-950. DOI: 10.1136/bjophthalmol-2013-304082. Epub 2014 Feb 13

[16] Fuller D, Machemer R, Knighton RW. Retinal damage produced by intraocular fiber optic light. American Journal of Ophthalmology. 1978;**85**(4):519-537. DOI: 10.1016/s0002-9394(14)75250-x

[17] Fishman GA, Anderson RJ, Lourenco P. Prevalence of posterior subcapsular lens opacities in patients with retinitis pigmentosa. The British Journal of Ophthalmology. 1985;**69**(4):263-266. DOI: 10.1136/bjo.69.4.263

[18] Chatterjee S, Agrawal D, Agrawal D, Parchand SM, Sahu A. Cataract surgery in retinitis pigmentosa. Indian Journal of Ophthalmology. 2021;**69**(7):1753-1757. DOI: 10.4103/ijo.IJO_2916_20

[19] Jin-Poi T, Shatriah I, Khairy-Shamel ST, Zunaina E. Rapid anterior capsular contraction after phacoemulsification surgery in a patient with retinitis pigmentosa. Clinical Ophthalmology. 2013;7:839-842. DOI: 10.2147/OPTH.S42122. Epub 2013 May 6

[20] Ascaso FJ, Huerva V, Grzybowski A. Epidemiology, etiology, and prevention of late IOL-capsular bag complex dislocation: Review of the literature. Journal of Ophthalmology. 2015;**2015**:805706. DOI: 10.1155/2015/805706. Epub 2015 Dec 21

[21] Lee BL, Sternberg JP. Microscope light toxicity. Sem Ophthalmology. 1993;**8**:151-155

[22] Nikpoor N, Stone DU. Rapid capsular phimosis in retinitis pigmentosa. Ophthalmic Surgery, Lasers & Imaging. 2010;**41**(6):e1-e3. DOI: 10.3928/15428877-20100726-12

[23] Sandberg MA, Brockhurst RJ, Gaudio AR, Berson EL. The association between visual acuity and central retinal thickness in retinitis pigmentosa. Investigative Ophthalmology & Visual Science. 2005;**46**(9):3349-3354. DOI: 10.1167/iovs.04-1383

[24] Aizawa S, Mitamura Y, Hagiwara A, Sugawara T, Yamamoto S. Changes of fundus autofluorescence, photoreceptor inner and outer segment junction line, and visual function in patients with retinitis pigmentosa. Clinical & Experimental Ophthalmology. 2010;**38**(6):597-604. DOI: 10.1111/j.1442-9071.2010.02321.x. Epub 2010 Apr 29

[25] Abe K, Iijima H, Hirakawa H, Tsukahara Y, Toda Y. Visual acuity and 10 degrees automated static perimetry in eyes with retinitis pigmentosa. Japanese Journal of Ophthalmology. 2002;**46**(5):581-585. DOI: 10.1016/s0021-5155(02)00548-8

[26] Hagiwara A, Yamamoto S, Ogata K, Sugawara T, Hiramatsu A, Shibata M, et al. Macular abnormalities in patients with retinitis pigmentosa: Prevalence on OCT examination and outcomes of vitreoretinal surgery. Acta Ophthalmologica. 2011;**89**(2):e122-e125. DOI: 10.1111/j.1755-3768.2010.01866.x

[27] Fishman GA, Fishman M, Maggiano J. Macular lesions associated with retinitis pigmentosa. Archives of Ophthalmology. 1977;**95**(5):798-803. DOI: 10.1001/archopht.1977.04450050076006

[28] Bu SC, Kuijer R, Li XR, Hooymans JM, Los LI. Idiopathic epiretinal membrane. Retina. 2014;**34**(12):2317-2335. DOI: 10.1097/IAE.0000000000000349

[29] dell'Omo R, Virgili G, Rizzo S, De Turris S, Coclite G, Giorgio D, et al. Role of lamellar hole-associated epiretinal proliferation in lamellar macular holes. American Journal of Ophthalmology. 2017;**175**:16-29. DOI: 10.1016/j.ajo.2016.11.007. Epub 2016 Nov 24

[30] Pang CE, Spaide RF, Freund KB. Comparing functional and morphologic characteristics of lamellar macular holes with and without lamellar hole-associated epiretinal proliferation. Retina. 2015;**35**(4):720-726. DOI: 10.1097/IAE.0000000000000390

[31] Vingolo EM, Valente S, Gerace E, Spadea L, Nebbioso M. Macular hole in retinitis pigmentosa patients: Microincision vitrectomy with polydimethylsiloxane as possible treatment. Eye (London, England). 2015;**29**(5):699-702. DOI: 10.1038/eye.2014.344. Epub 2015 Feb 20

[32] Iovino C, Rosolia A, Damiano L, Iodice CM, Di Iorio V, Testa F, et al. Pars Plana vitrectomy in inherited retinal diseases: A comprehensive review of the literature. Life (Basel). 2023;**13**(6):1241. DOI: 10.3390/life13061241

[33] Mishra K, Scott AW. Management of vitreomacular traction. In: Albert DM, Miller JW, Azar DT, Young LH, editors. Albert and Jakobiec's Principles and Practice of Ophthalmology. Cham: Springer; 2022. DOI: 10.1007/978-3-030-42634-7_104

[34] Johnson MW. Posterior vitreous detachment: Evolution and complications of its early stages. American Journal of Ophthalmology. 2010;**149**(3):371-82.e1. DOI: 10.1016/j.ajo.2009.11.022

[35] Ikeda Y, Yoshida N, Murakami Y, Nakatake S, Notomi S, Hisatomi T, et al. Long-term surgical outcomes of epiretinal membrane in patients with retinitis pigmentosa. Scientific Reports. 2015;**5**:13078. DOI: 10.1038/srep13078

[36] Yan F, Xia FJ, Jiang F, Yu HG. Visual and morphological outcomes of vitreomacular traction syndrome in retinitis pigmentosa treated by vitrectomy. International Journal of Ophthalmology. 2018;**11**(8):1411-1415. DOI: 10.18240/ijo.2018.08.25

[37] Vingolo EM, Gerace E, Valente S, Spadea L, Nebbioso M. Microincision vitrectomy surgery in vitreomacular traction syndrome of retinitis pigmentosa patients. BioMed Research International. 2014;**2014**:537081. DOI: 10.1155/2014/537081. Epub 2014 Jun 9

[38] Jin ZB, Gan DK, Xu GZ, Nao-I N. Macular hole formation in patients with retinitis pigmentosa and prognosis of pars plana vitrectomy. Retina. 2008;**28**(4):610-614. DOI: 10.1097/IAE.0b013e31815ec341

[39] García-Fernández M, Castro-Navarro J, Bajo-Fuente A.

Unilateral recurrent macular hole in a patient with retinitis pigmentosa: A case report. Journal of Medical Case Reports. 2013;7:69. DOI: 10.1186/1752-1947-7-69

[40] Lee CY, Yang CM, Yang CH, Hu FR, Chen TC. Flap technique-assisted surgeries for advanced retinitis pigmentosa complicated with macular hole: A case report and literature review. BMC Ophthalmology. 2021;**21**(1):322. DOI: 10.1186/s12886-021-02082-3

[41] Mahmoud TH, McCuen BW 2nd, Hao Y, Moon SJ, Tatebayashi M, Stinnett S, et al. Lensectomy and vitrectomy decrease the rate of photoreceptor loss in rhodopsin P347L transgenic pigs. Graefe's Archive for Clinical and Experimental Ophthalmology. 2003;**241**(4):298-308. DOI: 10.1007/s00417-003-0637-5. Epub 2003 Mar 21

[42] Coppola M, Cicinelli MV, Rabiolo A, Querques G, Bandello F. Importance of light filters in modern vitreoretinal surgery: An update of the literature. Ophthalmic Research. 2017;**58**(4):189-193. DOI: 10.1159/000475760. Epub 2017 Jun 2

[43] Miura G, Baba T, Yamamoto S. Two cases with retinitis pigmentosa that developed severe retinal atrophy long after vitreo-retinal surgery. American Journal of Ophthalmology Case Reports. 2020;**18**:100716. DOI: 10.1016/j.ajoc.2020.100716

[44] Gandorfer A, Haritoglou C, Kampik A. Toxicity of indocyanine green in vitreoretinal surgery. Developments in Ophthalmology. 2008;**42**:69-81. DOI: 10.1159/000138974

[45] Irigoyen C, Amenabar Alonso A, Sanchez-Molina J, Rodríguez-Hidalgo M, Lara-López A, Ruiz-Ederra J. Subretinal injection techniques for retinal disease: A review. Journal of Clinical Medicine. 12 Aug 2022;**11**(16):4717. DOI: 10.3390/jcm11164717

[46] Peng Y, Tang L, Zhou Y. Subretinal injection: A review on the novel route of therapeutic delivery for vitreoretinal diseases. Ophthalmic Research. 2017;**58**:217-226

[47] Russell S, Bennett J, Wellman JA, Chung DC, Yu ZF, Tillman A, et al. Efficacy and safety of voretigene neparvovec (AAV2-hRPE65v2) in patients with RPE65-mediated inherited retinal dystrophy: A randomised, controlled, open-label, phase 3 trial. Lancet. 2017;**390**(10097):849-860. DOI: 10.1016/S0140-6736(17)31868-8. Epub 2017 Jul 14. Erratum in: Lancet. 2017 Aug 26;390(10097):848. doi: 10.1016/S0140-6736(17)32235-3

[48] Koponen S, Kokki E, Kinnunen K, Ylä-Herttuala S. Viral-vector-delivered anti-angiogenic therapies to the eye. Pharmaceutics. 2021;**13**(2):219. DOI: 10.3390/pharmaceutics13020219

[49] Varela-Fernández R, Díaz-Tomé V, Luaces-Rodríguez A, Conde-Penedo A, García-Otero X, Luzardo-Álvarez A, et al. Drug delivery to the posterior segment of the eye: Biopharmaceutic and pharmacokinetic considerations. Pharmaceutics. 2020;**12**:269

[50] Park SW, Kim JH, Park WJ, Kim JH. Limbal approach-subretinal injection of viral vectors for gene therapy in mice retinal pigment epithelium. Journal of Visualized Experiments. 2015;**102**:e53030. DOI: 10.3791/53030

[51] Fan KC, Yannuzzi NA, Patel NA, Negron CI, Sisk RA, Nagiel A, et al. Surgical techniques for the subretinal delivery of pediatric gene therapy. Ophthalmology Retina. 2020;**4**(6):644-645. DOI: 10.1016/j.oret.2020.01.023. Epub 2020 Feb 5

[52] Xue K, Groppe M, Salvetti AP, MacLaren RE. Technique of retinal gene therapy: Delivery of viral vector into the subretinal space. Eye (London, England). 2017;**31**(9):1308-1316. DOI: 10.1038/eye.2017.158. Epub 2017 Aug 18

[53] Bainbridge JW, Smith AJ, Barker SS, Robbie S, Henderson R, Balaggan K, et al. Effect of gene therapy on visual function in Leber's congenital amaurosis. The New England Journal of Medicine. 2008;**358**(21):2231-2239. DOI: 10.1056/NEJMoa0802268. Epub 2008 Apr 27

[54] Fischer MD, Hickey DG, Singh MS, MacLaren RE. Evaluation of an optimized injection system for retinal gene therapy in human patients. Human Gene Therapy Methods. 2016;**27**(4):150-158. DOI: 10.1089/hgtb.2016.086

[55] Jacobson SG, Acland GM, Aguirre GD, Aleman TS, Schwartz SB, Cideciyan AV, et al. Safety of recombinant adeno-associated virus type 2-RPE65 vector delivered by ocular subretinal injection. Molecular Therapy. 2006;**13**(6):1074-1084. DOI: 10.1016/j.ymthe.2006.03.005. Epub 2006 Apr 27

[56] MacLaren RE, Groppe M, Barnard AR, Cottriall CL, Tolmachova T, Seymour L, et al. Retinal gene therapy in patients with choroideremia: Initial findings from a phase 1/2 clinical trial. Lancet. 2014;**383**(9923):1129-1137. DOI: 10.1016/S0140-6736(13)62117-0. Epub 2014 Jan 16

[57] Sastry A, Li JD, Raynor W, Viehland C, Song Z, Xu L, et al. Microscope-integrated OCT-guided volumetric measurements of subretinal blebs created by a suprachoroidal approach. Translational Vision Science & Technology. 2021;**10**:24

[58] Simunovic MP, Xue K, Jolly JK, MacLaren RE. Structural and functional recovery following limited iatrogenic macular detachment for retinal gene therapy. JAMA Ophthalmology. 2017;**135**(3):234-241. DOI: 10.1001/jamaophthalmol.2016.5630

Chapter 8

Penetrating Keratoplasty as an Inevitable Technique of Keratoplasty: Indications, Surgical Technique, and Outcomes

Mathew Shemiakin and Gulzhiyan Arzhimatova

Abstract

Today, keratoplasty technologies have developed greatly. Despite the widespread use of layered corneal surgery techniques, penetrating corneal transplantation remains the method of choice in many clinical cases. To a certain extent, it can be said that penetrating keratoplasty is performed on patients who had an unsuccessful experience with layered corneal transplantations. In other cases, penetrating corneal transplantation is required for patients who have contraindications to layered procedures: corneal ulcer with a risk of perforation or perforation, corneal thinning (less than 200 μm), severe vascularization, and corneal leukoma. In this chapter, the authors tried to highlight clinical situations in which penetrating keratoplasty is the only way to save the eye. Modern concepts of the pathogenetic mechanisms of penetrating corneal transplant disease are explained. Current techniques that help reduce the incidence of corneal transplant disease are described in detail. Clinical cases are presented as examples of the management of patients with penetrating corneal transplant disease during high-risk operations.

Keywords: high-risk penetrating keratoplasty (PK), corneal transplant disease, urgent penetrate keratoplasty, ulcer cornea with perforation, neovascularization of penetrating corneal transplant

1. Introduction

Nowadays, lamellar corneal surgery techniques are undergoing rapid development. An increasing number of surgeons are turning to lamellar keratoplasty methods (anterior and posterior automated keratoplasty using a femtosecond laser), as well as to procedures involving intrastromal segments to strengthen the corneal stroma in cases of keratoconus.

The first description of a posterior lamellar keratoplasty technique appeared in the literature in 1956 when C.W. Tillet performed a transplantation of the corneal endothelium and the posterior layers of the stroma [1]. According to the Eye Bank Association of America (EBAA), in 2009, posterior lamellar keratoplasty accounted for 45% of all keratoplasties performed for endothelial corneal pathology in the

United States; by 2011 and 2012, this procedure was used three times more frequently than penetrating keratoplasty for the treatment of endothelial dystrophies. One of the main reasons for this shift in favor of lamellar corneal surgery is the belief that penetrating keratoplasty is one of the most traumatic surgeries, carrying a high risk of severe intra- and postoperative complications such as graft disease, post-keratoplasty glaucoma, postoperative inflammation, intraoperative expulsive hemorrhage, and membrane detachment, as well as significant postoperative astigmatism.

From a historical perspective, the first successful outcomes of penetrating keratoplasty were achieved with small-diameter grafts (2–4 mm). This operation was termed "partial penetrating keratoplasty". Transplantation of a large-diameter corneal graft (more than 5 mm) is known as subtotal penetrating keratoplasty. The first instance of achieving a clear graft with a large-diameter transplant was demonstrated by N.A. Puchkovskaya (1950–1954), a student of V.P. Filatov. Widespread successful replacement of large corneal discs became possible only after the emergence of microsurgical techniques and ultrafine atraumatic suture materials. Microsurgical techniques and a large open approach to the eye cavity made it possible to combine the capabilities of keratoplasty and intraocular surgery into a single procedure. This led to a new direction in ophthalmic surgery—reconstruction of the anterior and posterior segments of the eye by means of open surgical access provided by extensive corneal trephination. In such cases, keratoplasty is often performed in combination with other interventions, such as dissection of synechiae and restoration of the anterior chamber, removal of dense membrane-like formations, iris reconstruction and pupil repositioning, cataract extraction and intraocular lens implantation, vitrectomy, and removal of a luxated lens and foreign bodies, among others.

When performing subtotal penetrating keratoplasty involving a large trephination opening in the cornea, proper anesthetic management (with a preference for general anesthesia), controlled intraoperative hypotension, and extremely careful surgical manipulation are all essential. Even slight muscle tension or irregular breathing on the part of the patient can lead to lens dislocation into the wound or other severe hemorrhagic complications. Therefore, this procedure is performed under general anesthesia in children and restless adults.

Keratoplasty is part of the broader biological problem of organ and tissue transplantation. It should be noted that the cornea is a fortunate exception among other transplantable tissues. Due to the absence of blood vessels and its separation from the eye's vascular tract by the intraocular fluid, the cornea has a relatively isolated immune status, allowing successful keratoplasty without strict donor-recipient matching. Currently, the most favorable and long-lasting graft survival following penetrating keratoplasty is observed in patients with keratoconus (12–20 years, with a survival rate of 90–100%). In patients with epithelial-endothelial corneal dystrophy, this rate is 51.7% [2]. It must be emphasized that the duration of graft transparency largely depends on endothelial health. Donor graft endothelial cell density gradually decreases over the course of 20 years post-transplantation, with an associated increase in the coefficient of variation in cell size and corneal thickness and a decrease in the percentage of hexagonal cells. Grafts with insufficient endothelial cell counts are prone to late endothelial failure, the primary reason for graft rejection within the first 5 years after surgery [3].

In light of the above, there has been a noticeable increase in the number of patients who have previously undergone lamellar corneal procedures and require repeat keratoplasty. Many authors use the term "high-risk keratoplasty" in their publications to describe patients with a predictably high risk of graft failure [4–9]. This high-risk category also includes patients with vascularized corneal opacities, ulcers with perforation, and corneal abscesses; for such patients, "high-risk" penetrating keratoplasty is often the only chance to save the eye and restore vision. In these emergency cases, surgery is performed during an active inflammatory phase in an attempt to prevent severe complications—uveitis, endophthalmitis, or panophthalmitis—that can lead to vision loss. Under these circumstances, graft survival rates 3 years after repeat corneal transplantation vary from 28 to 81% [10, 11].

2. When does penetrating keratoplasty become the last chance to save the eye?

Often, patients with inflammatory corneal conditions unresponsive to conservative treatment arrive at the emergency department and require urgent penetrating keratoplasty for tectonic or therapeutic purposes. These cases can be divided into two groups:

1. Corneal ulcers with perforation (perforation diameter greater than 2 mm).

2. Deep corneal ulcers with a risk of perforation.

In both groups, corneal pathology develops against the backdrop of active inflammation (keratitis) caused by various etiological factors. In young people who wear soft contact lenses improperly, an aggressive inflammatory process is often provoked by contamination with a microorganism—or a group of microorganisms—leading to treatment difficulties, a protracted course, and complications such as corneal ulcer perforation with subsequent need for tectonic keratoplasty.

Not infrequently, mechanical trauma to the corneal epithelium followed by secondary fungal infection can occur after a course of antibacterial therapy. Fungal corneal infiltrates require extended (more than 3 months) systemic and topical treatment. Delayed therapy may cause the infection to spread into the anterior chamber of the eye, resulting in uveitis. If the fungi spread to the ciliary body, treatment becomes significantly more challenging, and prognosis worsens since eradicating fungi from the choroid is no trivial task. In such cases, therapeutic keratoplasty is indicated.

For patients in the above groups, penetrating keratoplasty is often the only chance to save the eye. The rate of graft complications and rejection varies depending on the type of keratoplasty. Penetrating keratoplasty has a rejection rate of about 29%, with endothelial rejection being the most common type [12]. In the long term, rejection and endothelial failure are the primary causes of penetrating keratoplasty failure, with a graft survival rate of approximately 73.5% at 5 years under systemic immunosuppression [13]. In patients with glaucoma, especially those who have undergone previous surgeries, the rejection risk is significantly higher, reaching up to 35% at 10 years [14]. In children undergoing therapeutic keratoplasty, the rejection rate stands at around 12.1%, and the success rate of treatment is lower due to delays in initiating therapy [15]. During therapeutic keratoplasty, the risk of rejection increases because inflammation or perforation is frequently present at the time of surgery. Overall rejection rates range from 30 to 40% [16]. This is due to the immunocytochemical environment encountered by the donor endothelium. A high titer of proinflammatory cytokines in the anterior chamber fluid and the pharmacological load (antibacterial, antiseptic, and antifungal treatment) used to combat the infection can exhaust the donor endothelium. Its failure results in chronic hypoxia and the growth of neovascularization [11]. This neovascularization closes the loop of graft disease, leading to graft opacity and the necessity for repeat penetrating keratoplasty.

3. Surgical techniques of penetrating keratoplasty: When no universal algorithm exists

The requirements for donor tissue in penetrating keratoplasty are significantly higher than for lamellar procedures. This is because a penetrating graft contains all the layers of the cornea, including one particularly sensitive to changing conditions: the single-layer endothelium (sometimes referred to as the "posterior epithelium"), which has a unique, glial-type origin. These endothelial cells are always the first to die and cannot fully regenerate. After surgery, all donor corneal structures are gradually replaced by the recipient's corneal tissue—except for the endothelial cells, which continue to survive and ensure the viability of the entire graft. For this reason, penetrating keratoplasty is sometimes referred to as the art of transplanting a single row of endothelial cells. This explains both the strict quality requirements for donor tissue in penetrating keratoplasty and the need for utmost care when handling the cornea's posterior surface during surgery.

For penetrating keratoplasty, a cadaveric cornea obtained no more than 24 hours postmortem is typically used. In some clinics, donor corneas are preserved in specialized media, and these preservation techniques continue to evolve. Donor tissue is rigorously tested for HIV, hepatitis, and other infections. Biomicroscopy of the donor's eye is also performed to rule out any pathological changes in the cornea and to identify possible consequences of prior anterior segment surgeries.

Penetrating keratoplasty as a procedure is over a century old. Originally introduced by Eduard Zirm, it has spawned numerous modifications, though the core technique has changed relatively little. In the operating room, a corneal button of 8.0–9.0 mm in diameter—usually 0.25 mm larger than the recipient bed—is trephined from a pre-prepared donor corneoscleral button. Trephination and subsequent excision of the recipient's corneal tissue are performed with at least a 0.25 mm margin beyond the affected corneal area, followed by suturing of the pre-cut donor graft in place. The graft is secured using interrupted and/or running 10-0 nylon sutures in the prepared recipient bed. Balanced Salt Solution (BSS) is then introduced into the recipient's anterior chamber until normal intraocular pressure is achieved, concluding the procedure.

However, "high-risk" penetrating keratoplasty is not a standard operation. In most cases, this is because the surgeon may encounter intraoperative "surprises," circumstances that cannot always be anticipated—even with considerable surgical experience.

3.1 What size donor graft should be used?

Depending on the size of the donor graft, the penetrating keratoplasty is divided into the following types:

- Partial—up to 5 mm.
- Subtotal—from 5 to 9 mm.
- Total—more than 9 mm.

When performing the operation, surgeons, when choosing the size of the donor transplant, are guided by the size of the pathological focus of the affected cornea. In the presence of an ulcerative defect, infiltrate, or opacity zone requiring penetrating keratoplasty, it is advisable to perform trepanation of the damaged tissue of the recipient's cornea with the capture of healthy tissue by 0.25 mm. For patients with vascularized leukomas, dystrophy of the entire thickness of the cornea, and other clinical situations requiring penetrating keratoplasty, the surgeon has the opportunity to choose the size of the trepanation bed. A number of surgeons perform the operation using a donor transplant similar in diameter to the size of the recipient's trepanation. For partial and subtotal keratoplasty, this gives a good result.

For patients in the "high-risk" keratoplasty group with a diagnosis of ulcer with perforation and corneal infiltrate, the surgeon has to use trephines with a diameter greater than the size of the perforation or infiltrate by 0.25–0.5 mm. In such cases, there is a high need to perform total keratoplasty with suturing of the limbus area. It should be taken into account that in the postoperative period, against the background of active inflammation in the structures of the anterior chamber angle, the formation of synechia and the development of secondary ophthalmic hypertension is possible.

3.2 Which sutures provide the best graft fixation?

In global practice, 10-0 nylon sutures are commonly used to secure the donor cornea to the recipient tissue. Some specialists place 10-0 nylon interrupted "guide" sutures, then remove them after placing and tightening a continuous (running) 10-0 nylon "encircling" suture. There are also techniques involving two continuous running sutures, which, according to some authors, help reduce postoperative astigmatism.

It is important to note that in cases of graft fixation for patients with corneal ulcers and infiltrates undergoing surgery against a background of active inflammation, the continuous 10-0 nylon suture may sometimes cut through the friable tissue. This can lead to wound edge dehiscence and necessitate additional interrupted sutures. Placing 16–24 interrupted 10-0 nylon sutures can significantly reduce the likelihood of postoperative suture cut-through when the corneal tissue is compromised.

In extreme cases of pronounced suture cut-through, the surgeon may opt for a thicker 9-0 nylon suture. Although this is not standard practice, it can ensure reliable fixation of the penetrating graft in urgent or difficult situations.

3.3 When should the lens be removed?

There are two prevailing opinions on this issue. The first suggests that the lens should be removed during keratoplasty; the second maintains that the lens should be preserved. Proponents of each view present their own arguments.

Those favoring lens removal argue that during inflammation, the anterior chamber fluid contains a significant amount of proinflammatory cytokines capable of affecting the lens. This can cause lens swelling and result in secondary ocular hypertension due to the closure of the anterior chamber angle. A subsequent intervention would expose the donor endothelium to additional trauma, increasing the likelihood of graft-related complications.

Another group of surgeons believes that the native lens serves a barrier function in the presence of inflammation in the cornea, iris, and anterior chamber fluid, preventing the spread of inflammation to the posterior segment of the eye. Moreover, combining corneal grafting with cataract extraction on an "open sky" eye significantly increases the scope of surgery and the risk of expulsive complications.

In practice, each clinical situation is unique. The decision regarding the extent of surgery is made either by the surgeon or through a multidisciplinary consultation.

However, every action must be justified, and the benefits of intraoperative manipulations should outweigh the potential risks.

3.4 What scope of reconstruction should be performed?

The goal of reconstruction is to create anatomically favorable conditions for both the eye and the donor graft. For patients needing penetrating keratoplasty (PKP) for a perforated corneal ulcer or corneal infiltrate, the extent of reconstruction depends on various factors.

If the iris is plugging the corneal defect (e.g., by forming an iris tamponade), it should be separated from the affected tissue, with a decision then made regarding whether iris excision or iridoplasty is indicated, based on the iris's viability. When the process is located near the limbal area and involves the anterior chamber angle and iris root, reconstruction of the anterior chamber angle and dissection of anterior goniosynechiae are required.

If the pupil is adherent to the anterior lens capsule or the iris is bowed forward (bombé), a peripheral iridotomy in at least two quadrants should be performed intraoperatively. In the video example mentioned, one can see how challenging it can be to separate the affected tissue from the iris and reconstruct the anterior chamber angle in patients who have already undergone multiple penetrating keratoplasties.

Regardless, when performing penetrating keratoplasty, the reconstruction should be as minimally traumatic as possible while still being maximally effective.

3.5 How to conclude the surgery: Air, BSS, or something else?

After replacing the diseased cornea with donor tissue, completing the reconstruction, and placing a continuous suture, the surgeon must decide what to leave in the anterior chamber at the end of the operation.

Under standard circumstances—for instance, when performing keratoplasty for keratoconus or other degenerative-dystrophic conditions—filling the anterior chamber with sterile Balanced Salt Solution (BSS) is generally recommended because its composition is closest to the natural aqueous humor. BSS is also easily replaced postoperatively by the patient's own aqueous humor, causing minimal discomfort.

In certain situations, if there is leakage of aqueous humor through corneal incisions, surgeons may use sterile air due to its higher surface tension, which can help maintain anterior chamber integrity in the early postoperative period. However, the presence of air in the anterior chamber requires that the patient maintain a specific head position after surgery. If the air bubble shifts into the posterior chamber, iridocorneal contact may develop, leading to increased intraocular pressure. This scenario might necessitate further intervention.

Unfortunately, using viscoelastics (cohesive, adhesive, or others) as a fill for the anterior chamber at the end of surgery has no clear advantages. In some cases, they can obstruct outflow pathways and contribute to elevated intraocular pressure; in others, they create conditions favoring inflammation in the postoperative period.

3.6 Clinical cases

In order to illustrate the various challenges a specialist performing penetrating keratoplasty may encounter, let us consider several clinical cases.

3.6.1 Case 1

A 33-year-old patient diagnosed with an infectious corneal infiltrate presented to the emergency ophthalmology department with complaints of decreased vision in the right eye (OD), tearing, photophobia, and pain for 30 days. These symptoms first appeared after swimming in the ocean. The patient had been treated for a month with dexamethasone and antibiotics. Visual acuity: OD = pr. l. incerta; OS = 1.0; IOP in both eyes was noted as "normal." A drawing of the right eye can be seen in **Figure 1**.

The patient underwent penetrating keratoplasty aimed at preserving the integrity of the eye. Early in the postoperative period, hypopyon was detected, and the anterior chamber was irrigated multiple times with antibiotic solutions. On the seventh day, microbiological culture results identified Fusarium species, prompting the initiation of active antifungal therapy. After 30 days of intensive treatment, the patient's cataract began to swell, and secondary ocular hypertension developed. Consequently, extracapsular cataract extraction was performed.

Despite continued antibacterial therapy, the patient returned 90 days after the initial operation with complaints of reduced vision and pain in the affected eye. The ophthalmic findings at that time are shown in **Figure 2**.

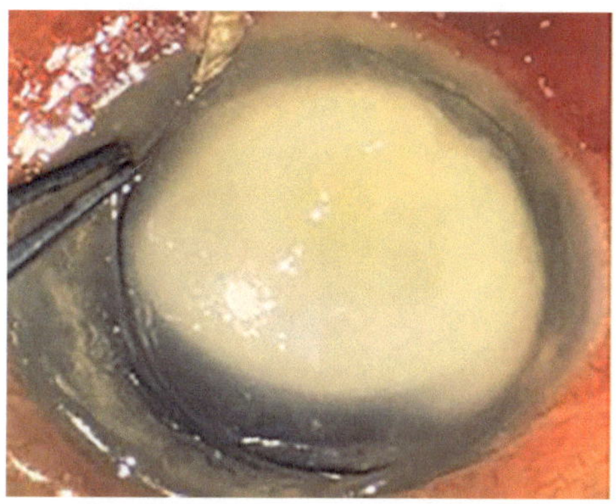

Figure 1.
Corneal infiltrate with a diameter of 9 mm. Photo from the operating room.

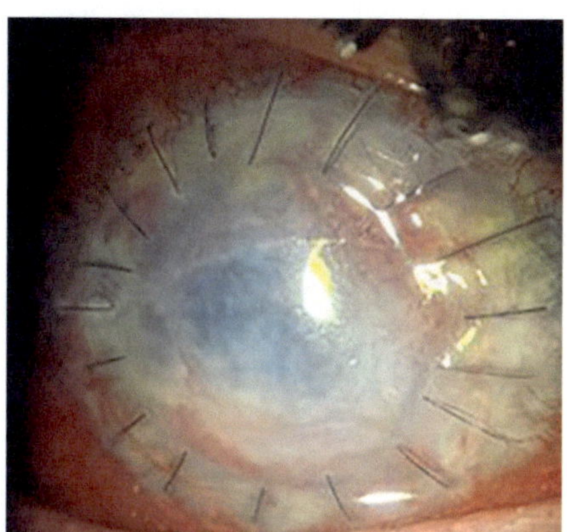

Figure 2.
Graft disease, neovascularization, shallow anterior chamber, aphakia. Condition 3 months after the first penetrating keratoplasty.

Taking into account the patient's young age, the absence of significant posterior segment pathology, and the patient's strong desire to preserve vision, a decision was made to perform repeat keratoplasty with reconstruction of the anterior chamber angle. Video 2 (https://drive.google.com/drive/folders/1yzBlFTBLRrms mH1QRrERTY7KUJLGsUpn) illustrates the delicate process of separating fibrous tissue in the anterior segment of the eye, including iris stabilization, iridotomy, release of the anterior chamber angle structures, and removal of posterior hyaloid fibrosis. Three months of ongoing anti-inflammatory and antifungal treatment followed, and the condition of the graft after this period is demonstrated in **Figures 3** and **4**.

3.6.2 Case 2

Patient R, 54 years old, presented to the emergency department with complaints of redness, pain, and decreased vision in the left eye. According to the history,

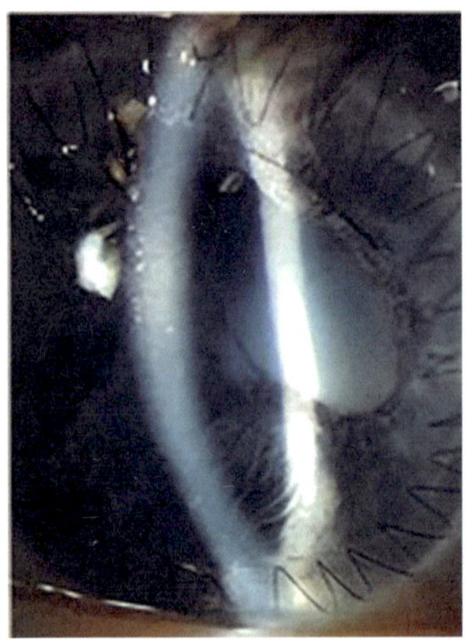

Figure 3.
The cornea is transparent, with chamber of medium depth, anterior-chamber moisture without inflammation.

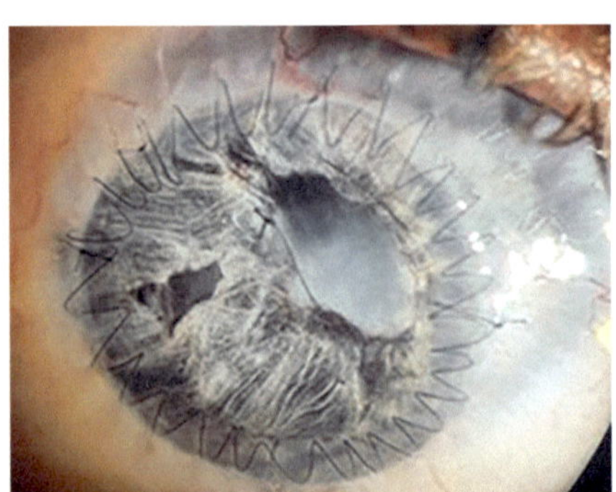

Figure 4.
The cornea is transparent, slight fibrosis of the posterior capsule is visible, and the sutures on the corneas are clean and consistent.

these symptoms began 1 month ago. He was treated at a regional hospital with a diagnosis of keratouveitis (OS) but showed no improvement. Treatment included topical aminoglycosides and fluoroquinolone, as well as systemic glycopeptides (vancomycin 1 g twice a day) for 7 days. The ophthalmic findings are shown in **Figure 5**.

Due to the lack of response to antibacterial therapy, the patient underwent organ-preserving penetrating keratoplasty. Video 3 illustrates the surgical procedure. An intraoperative culture was taken, and after 4 days, the results indicated the growth of *Fusarium solani* at 10^1 CFU/ml (**Figure 6**). In the early postoperative period, the patient received both antibacterial and antifungal therapies. **Figure 7** shows the condition of the eye 14 days post-surgery.

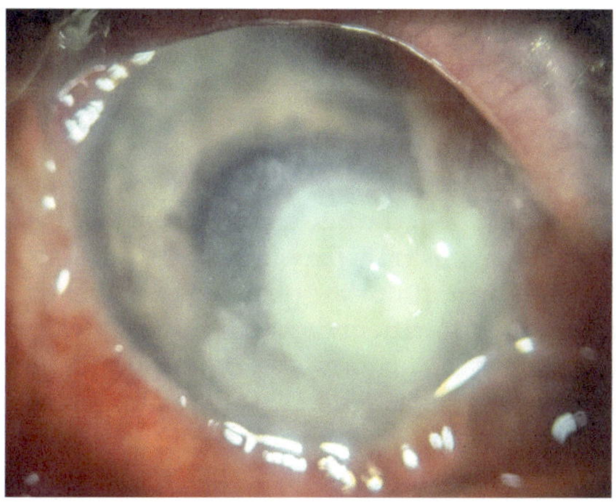

Figure 5.
Mixed injection of the conjunctiva. Edematous dull cornea, in the lower half with involvement of the optical zone there is an extensive infiltrate with an expression.

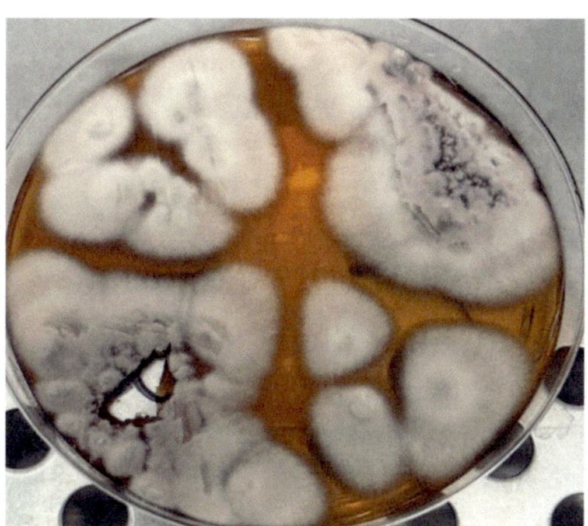

Figure 6.
Macroscopically extracted mushroom cultures on a Petri dish.

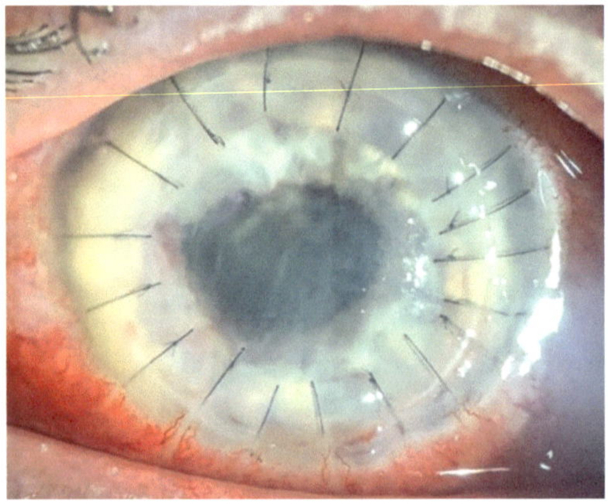

Figure 7.
The nodal sutures on the cornea are clean and consistent. Moisture in the anterior chamber is transparent.

4. Outcomes of penetrating keratoplasty

It is widely recognized that penetrating keratoplasty (PK) has two possible outcomes: either the graft remains transparent, or "graft disease" ensues. Maintaining graft transparency depends on appropriate postoperative therapy, timely adjunctive interventions, and a high level of patient compliance. The lifespan of a corneal graft largely depends on the underlying diagnosis, spanning approximately 10–15 years for "low-risk" penetrating keratoplasties and 3–5 years for "high-risk" groups. "Graft disease" refers to loss of transparency in the postoperative period, resulting from either immunologic or non-immunologic factors. Manifestations may include immunologic rejection of any corneal layer, recurrence or onset of a new infectious process on the graft, a trophic ulcer leading to perforation, graft neovascularization, endothelial failure, and stromal edema with consequent opacity. A primary question posed by patients facing "high-risk" penetrating keratoplasty concerns the likelihood of successful graft survival. Numerous authors have examined risk factors affecting graft longevity, consistently reporting higher rates of graft disease following PK compared to lamellar techniques. A recognized test—and a contraindication to surgery—is the "inhibition" of leukocyte migration in response to corneal antigens (the RTML assay), which indicates heightened cellular autoimmunity (a key factor in transplantation). Prior to keratoplasty, positive findings in this assay are detected with varying frequency (4–50%), depending on corneal disease etiology, clinical characteristics, treatment regimen, and other factors. A marked tissue-specific response in the first 2–3 weeks post-surgery is to be expected, but if "inhibition" in the RTML assay is noted at later stages, the risk of a biological graft response rises substantially. Additional insights can be gained by observing changes in the ratio of immunoregulatory T-cell subpopulations: progressive increases in $CD4^+$ cells alongside decreases in $CD8^+$ cells (thus elevating the CD4/CD8 index) favor systemic autoimmune processes. Testing for corneal-specific antibodies (via passive hemagglutination, RPHA) is generally uninformative, likely due to the formation of immune complexes with autoantigen.

Evaluating cytokine levels is critical for predicting keratoplasty outcomes and guiding immunosuppressive therapy. Pre- and postoperative detection of IL-1β and/

or TNFα in tear fluid or serum is associated with an increased risk of graft disease (persistent corneal erosions, neovascularization). Immune-inflammatory mediators and autoimmune reaction modulators, notably IL-2 and IFN-γ, play a central role. Persistent systemic hyperproduction of these cytokines reduces favorable keratoplasty outcomes to one-third the rate observed in cases of moderate cytokine levels, justifying the use of agents that suppress IL-2 and IFN-γ. Even widely used selective immunosuppressants in transplantation (cyclosporine A, FK506) must be administered under strict supervision.

Most episodes of Descemet's Stripping Endothelial Keratoplasty (DSEK) rejection occur in the first year, whereas PK graft rejection can occur over a span of several years. Some authors conclude that rejection in DSEK primarily relates to graft- or surgery-specific risk factors, while in PK, it is more often linked to factors inherent to the recipient [17]. For example, risk factors for graft failure include chemical burns, uncontrolled inflammation, purulent infections, autoimmune diseases, low donor endothelial cell density, and intraoperative complications. Chronic infections—especially those caused by herpesviruses and hepatitis B or C—are also considered risk factors. Illustratively, in chronic HBsAg carriers, corneal graft rejection was observed four times more often than in uninfected individuals. The likelihood of reactivating latent infections is largely dependent on interferon status. An inability to produce sufficient interferons to safeguard against viral activation—especially under immunosuppression—negatively impacts keratoplasty outcomes. On the other hand, virus-induced hyperproduction of IFN-α and particularly IFN-γ, as seen in some patients with herpetic corneal ulcers and post-burn corneal opacities (occurring in about one in five patients and 1.5–2 times more frequently post-keratoplasty), also portends a poor prognosis. This is attributable to the capacity of interferons to enhance the expression of class I (IFN-α, IFN-β, IFN-γ) and class II (IFN-γ) HLA molecules and to stimulate IL-1 production and, consequently, IL-2 release—thus activating cytotoxic lymphocytes, autoimmune reactions, and ultimately graft rejection with resultant graft opacity. For these reasons, the active use of interferon therapy is contraindicated in corneal, as well as other organ and tissue, transplantation. Certain social factors, such as completion of higher education and entering into marriage, have also been noted [18]. However, the risk factors identified through regression models are often challenging to employ in clinical practice.

Accordingly, the authors have proposed a risk assessment scale for predicting graft disease in penetrating corneal transplantation (PCNTD), adapted to meet clinicians' needs (**Table 1**). This scale is based on data from patients undergoing "high-risk" penetrating keratoplasty [19].

4.1 Clinical example of applying the PCNTD scale

Our findings indicated that patients with a high PCNTD score faced a greater risk of graft disease (GD) and more frequently required organ-preserving penetrating keratoplasty. Managing patients according to the scale's criteria led to improved graft survival rates and a reduction in the total score. Below is a clinical example demonstrating how the scale is used in practice.

A 33-year-old patient, M., presented with complaints of no vision, pain, and tearing in the right eye. Symptoms had been present for 10 days and were associated with improper use of soft contact lenses. Examination of the right eye (**Figure 8**)

PCNTD scale		
Criterion	**Values**	**Score**
Recipient age (years)	<59	0
	60–74	1
	75 and more	2
Localization of ulcer, infiltrate/thinning relative to the optical zone of the recipient's cornea	<Ø3mm.	1
	Ø3-6 mm.	2
	> Ø6mm.	3
Ulcer/infiltrate/thinning diameter (mm)	<5	1
	6–9	2
	>10	3
Established etiologic factor (EF)	Yes	0
	No	1
Determination of sensitivity to AB drugs (If there is a Ministry of Defense)	Yes	0
	No	2
Hypopyon in the anterior chamber	No	0
	Yes	2
Preexisting epithelial vascularization corneas (quadrant)	No	0
	1	0
	2	1
	3	2
	4	3
Preexisting stromal - endothelial vascularization corneas (quadrant)	No	0
	1	2
	2	3
	3	4
	4	5
Associated ophthalmologic events (In anamnesis)	Glaucoma	2
	Uveitis	2
	Previous keratoplasty	2
	Herpetic keratitis	3
	Two or more of the above	6
Associated general somatic events (in anamnesis)	Arterial hypertension	1
	Chronic sinusitis	1
	Covid19 (postponed)	1
	Diabetes mellitus	1
	Two or more of the above	3

Table 1.
Factors of the corneal graft disease prediction scale and assigned points based on regression model coefficients (n = 120).

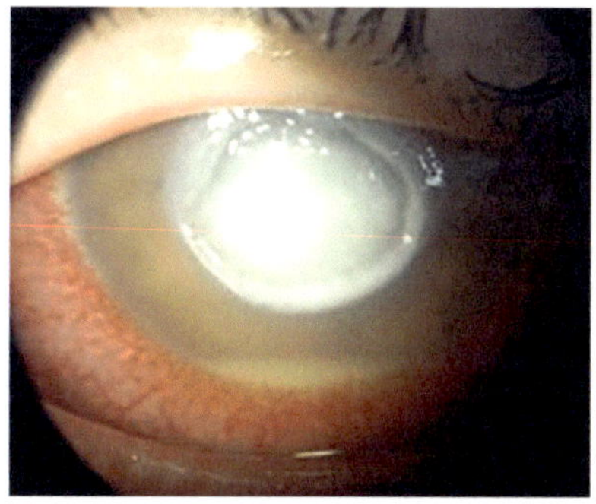

Figure 8.
Corneal ulcer to the deep layers of the stroma, 1 mm. hypopyon , uveitis, pericorneal injection.

showed an infectious corneal ulcer, uveitis, and a hypopyon. The PCNTD prognosis was calculated as follows:

- ulcer diameter of 6 mm = 2 points
- ulcer location within 3–6 mm of the optical zone = 2 points
- no identified microorganism and no established antibiotic sensitivity = 1 + 2 = 3 points
- hypopyon measuring 1 mm = 2 points
- presence of uveitis = 2 points
- chronic bilateral sinusitis and a previous COVID-19 infection in 2020 = 2 points

The total score according to the PCNTD scale was 13, corresponding to a moderate risk (35–37%) as per the regression equation data. In light of the lack of improvement with conservative therapy, the patient underwent penetrating keratoplasty (surgeon: G. Sh. Arzhimatova) with the dual aims of organ preservation and infection control. Postoperatively, the inflammatory process was brought under control, and sinusitis was treated adequately under the supervision of an ENT specialist (**Table 2**) [19].

However, on postoperative day 104, the graft became cloudy (**Figure 9**). Its condition did not improve with conservative treatment. Given the patient's young age, low

Risk of PCNTD (point)	Conditional probability of PCNTD (%)
Low (up to 7)	15.5
Average (8–13)	36.2
Tall (14–20)	62.3
Very high (21 and above)	>85.9

Table 2.
Stratification of patients at risk of graft disease depending on the score coefficient.

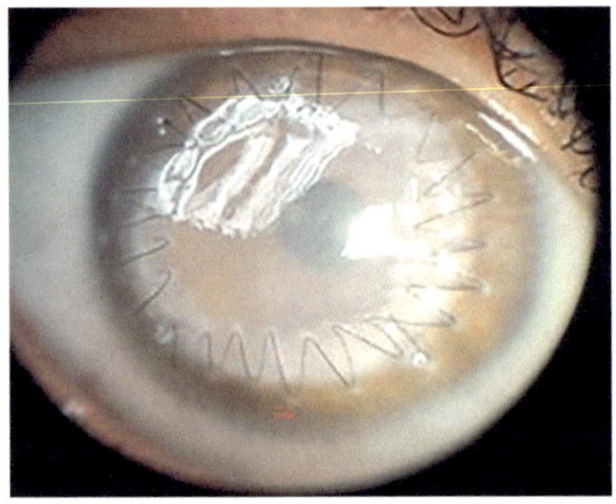

Figure 9.
Corneal graft edema, sutures are clean and well-maintained. There are no signs of uveitis after the course of therapy, 104 days after the PK.

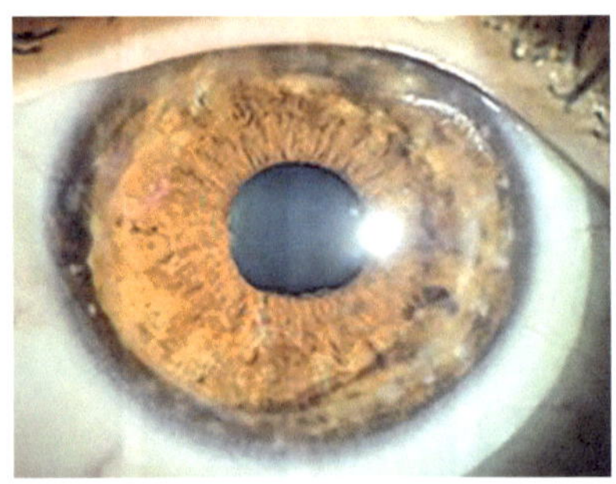

Figure 10.
The condition of the right eye cornea graft 24 months after penetrating second keratoplasty.

visual acuity, and the absence of deeper ocular pathology according to additional examinations, a decision was made to perform a repeat keratoplasty. Six months after the first surgery, a re-keratoplasty was carried out. Prior to this second procedure, the probability of GD was reassessed using the PCNTD scale. The patient scored 2 points for previously undergoing keratoplasty and 1 point for the 2020 COVID-19 infection, a total of 3 points—equivalent to a low (15.5%) risk of developing graft disease. Two years later, the transplant remains clear (**Figure 10**), and the sutures were removed 15 months postoperatively.

5. Conclusions

Despite significant advances in lamellar corneal surgery, penetrating keratoplasty remains a crucial procedure. In fact, the introduction of lamellar keratoplasty has contributed to the emergence of a sizable patient cohort requiring high-risk penetrating keratoplasty, largely due to multiple interventions on the same eye. Several clinical conditions—such as corneal ulcerations with perforation, corneal infiltrates, and vascularized corneal opacities—often mandate a "high-risk" keratoplasty approach. Worldwide, clinicians and researchers are endeavoring to elucidate the causes and risk factors associated with graft disease in patients undergoing penetrating keratoplasty. Achieving a successful outcome, namely the sustained transparency of the graft, necessitates a thorough exploration of the patient's medical history, a precise analysis of clinical findings, and an in-depth understanding of the pathogenesis of the underlying corneal pathology.

Intraoperatively, it is paramount to select an appropriate surgical strategy and determine the necessary extent of intervention. The operative approach should be minimally invasive yet maximally effective. Equally imperative is careful postoperative management: optimizing glucocorticosteroid therapy and initiating timely antibacterial and anti-inflammatory regimens are integral to preserving graft clarity. Retrospective analyses of clinical outcomes represent an essential facet of academic pursuits in major medical centers. Adapting these evidence-based insights to daily clinical practice is instrumental in safeguarding patient vision and advancing the field of corneal transplantation.

Acknowledgements

To the head of the Moscow Coordination Center for Organ Donation (MCCOD), Professor Doctor of Medical Sciences. Minina M.G., as well as employees of the bacteriological laboratory of the "Botkin Hospital" of the Moscow Department of Health, head of the laboratory Emelyanova E.B., bacteriologist Ugolnikova A.O.

Conflict of interest

The authors declare no conflict of interest.

Acronyms and abbreviations

PK	penetrating keratoplasty
GD	graft disease
IOP	intraocular pressure
RTML	reaction tissue migration leukocyte
CD 4	cluster of differentiation 4 type
CD 8	cluster of differentiation 8 type
IL-1β	interleukin-1 beta
TNFα	tumor necrosis factor alfa
IFN-γ	interferon gamma
DSEK	Descemet's stripping endothelial keratoplasty
HLA	human leucocyte antigens
PCNTD	penetrating corneal native transplant disease

Author details

Mathew Shemiakin[1*] and Gulzhiyan Arzhimatova[2]

1 Ophthalmologist of the Ophthalmological Department, Moscow City Ophthalmological Center (MCOC) "Botkin Hospital", Moscow, Russian Federation

2 Moscow State Medical Center, Moscow City Ophthalmological Center (MCOC) "Botkin Hospital", Moscow, Russian Federation

*Address all correspondence to: matvei.shemyakin@gmail.com

References

[1] Tillet CW. Posterior lamellar keratoplasty. American Journal of Ophthalmology. 1956;**41**(3):R.530-R.533

[2] Ono T, Ishiyama S, Hayashidera T, et al. Twelve-year follow-up of penetrating keratoplasty. Japanese Journal of Ophthalmology. 2017;**61**:131-136. DOI: 10.1007/s10384-016-0489-2

[3] Bourne WM. Cellular changes in transplanted human corneas. Cornea. 2001;**20**(6):560-569. DOI: 10.1097/00003226-200108000-00002

[4] Malyugin BE, Sakhnov SN, Myasnikova VV. Analysis of the results of end-to-end corneal transplantation in a retrospective cohort study. Ophthalmosurgery. 2021;**4**:12-20. DOI: 10.25276/0235-4160-2021-4-12-20. (in Russ.)

[5] Neroev VV, Balatskaya NV, Chentsova EV. Features of local and systemic production of pro-inflammatory, chemoattractant mediators and vascular growth factors in high-risk corneal transplants. Immunopathology, Allergology, Infectology. 2021;**1**:20-28. DOI: 10.14427/jipai.2021.1.20. (in Russ.)

[6] Mironkova EA, Demkin VV, Slepova OS. Diagnosis and role of HHV-6 infection in high-risk keratoplasty. Rossiyskiy Ophthalmologic Zhurnal. 2012;**5**(3):30-33. (in Russ.)

[7] Borzenok SA, Tonaeva KD, Onishchenko NA, Yu. Induction of local immune tolerance with the help of limbal cotransplantation in high-risk keratoplasty (literature review). Ophthalmosurgery. 2011;**2**:85-88. (in Russ.). Available from: https://eyepress.ru/article/induktsiya-lokal-noy-immunnoy-tolerantnosti-s-pomoshch-yu-limbal-noy-sotransplan

[8] Zazzo AD, Kheirkhah A, Abud TB, Goyal S, Dana R. Management of high risk corneal transplantation. Survey of Ophthalmology. 2017;**62**(6):816-827. DOI: 10.1016/j.survophthal.2016.12.010

[9] Armitage WJ, Goodchild C, Griffin MD, Gunn DJ, Hjortdal J, Lohan P, et al. High-risk corneal transplantation: Recent developments and future possibilities. Transplantation. 2019;**103**(12):2468-2478. DOI: 10.1097/TP.0000000000002938

[10] Dickman MM, Spekreijse LS, Dunker SL, Winkens B, Berendschot TTJM, van den Biggelaar FJHM, et al. Long-term outcomes of repeated corneal transplantations: A prospective Dutch registry study. American Journal of Ophthalmology. 2018;**193**:156-165. DOI: 10.1016/j.ajo.2018.06.018. Epub 2018 Jun 28

[11] Arzhimatova GS, Salikhov EA, Shemyakin MY. Corneal neovascularization: A modern view of molecular mechanisms and methods of therapy. Russian Ophthalmological Journal. 2023;**16**(2):153-159. DOI: 10.21516/2072-0076-2023-16-2-153-15. (in Russ.)

[12] Krachmer J. Clinical types of corneal transplant rejection. Their manifestations, frequency, preoperative correlates, and treatment. Archives of Ophthalmology. 1981;**99**(4):599-604. DOI: 10.1001/ARCHOPHT.1981.03930010599002

[13] Chow S, Cook S, Tole D. Long-term outcomes of high-risk

keratoplasty in patients receiving systemic immunosuppression. Cornea. 2015;**34**:1395-1399. DOI: 10.1097/ICO.0000000000000615

[14] Dunn S, Gal R, Kollman C, Raghinaru D, Dontchev M, Blanton C, et al. Corneal graft rejection 10 years after penetrating keratoplasty in the cornea donor study. Cornea. 2014;**33**:1003-1009. DOI: 10.1097/ICO.0000000000000212

[15] Kusumesh R, Vanathi M. Graft rejection in pediatric penetrating keratoplasty: Clinical features and outcomes. Oman Journal of Ophthalmology. 2015;**8**:33-37. DOI: 10.4103/0974-620X.149862

[16] Arzhimatova GS, Salikhov EA, Shemyakin MY, Ibraimov AI. Retrospective analysis of the results and causes of penetrating keratoplasty with native donor material in a multidisciplinary hospital (along the example of MCOC Botkin hospital). Ophthalmology in Russia. 2022;**19**(4):931-938. DOI: 10.18008/1816-5095-2022-4-931-938. (in Russ.)

[17] Duman F, Guler A, Kosker M, Azari AA, Marangoz D, Hammersmith KM, et al. A detailed analysis of individuals having graft failure after corneal transplantation. Seminars in Ophthalmology. 2024;**39**(8):634-638. DOI: 10.1080/08820538.2024.2354693. Epub 2024 May 16

[18] Yang Y, Zeng H, Gong L, Lin T. Risk factors for graft failure after penetrating keratoplasty in Eastern China from 2018 to 2021. Annals of Transplantation. 2024;**29**:e 945388. DOI: 10.12659/AOT.945388

[19] Arzhimatova GS, Chernakova GM, Salikhov EA, Shemyakin MY. Statistical analysis of risk factors in high-risk penetrating keratoplasty. Ophthalmology in Russia. 2024;**21**(3):509-516. (in Russ.). DOI: 10.18008/1816-5095-2024-3-509-516

Chapter 9

Efficacy and Safety Analysis of 0.01% and 0.05% Atropine Combined with OK Lens in Children with Progressive Myopia

Duo Xu, Yunyun Wang, Ling Ai, Benchu Feng, Zhilong Yang and Fuliang Li

Abstract

Myopia has become a global public health problem. With rising incidence rates among children and a trend toward earlier onset, treatment to slow the progression of myopia has become a quite important research area. Among them, orthokeratology (OK) lens is the first choice of myopia treatment for more and more adolescents because of its effectiveness in controlling myopia progression and the convenience of not needing to wear glasses during the day. However, it is worth noting that due to the diversity of myopia-affecting factors, there are still some adolescents with poor control effect. A number of studies have found that low-concentration atropine combined with OK lens can synergically enhance the myopia control effect in adolescents. In low-concentration atropine eye drops, the most commonly used concentrations are 0.01% and 0.05%. Therefore, this chapter reviews the efficacy and safety of 0.01% and 0.05% atropine eye drops in the combined use of OK lens in children with progressive myopia.

Keywords: 0.05% atropine, progressive myopia, myopia, effectiveness, adverse reactions

1. Introduction

Myopia has become a major global public health problem. According to the expert analysis of myopia epidemiology, it is predicted that by 2050, about 50% of the world's population will suffer from myopia, and up to 10% of the population will suffer from high myopia [1]. High myopia, especially pathological myopia, will lead to a series of eye complications, including retinal detachment, myopic macular degeneration, choroid neovascularization, cataracts, glaucoma, etc., which may eventually lead to permanent visual impairment [2]. As a result, treatments to slow the progression of myopia have become a fairly important area of research.

Currently recognized measures to control myopia are as follows: Atropine with different concentrations, OK lens, and defocusing glasses have all achieved varying degrees of myopia control effect in clinical practice [3], among which OK lens has been widely used in clinical practice due to its good control effect. OK lens is a specially designed rigid breathable contact lens that exerts pressure through the lens and the tear film underneath it, and thus temporarily changing the geometry of the cornea. After overnight wearing, the naked eye can maintain clear vision for 1 day during the day, and myopic defocus can be formed around the retina to effectively control the development of myopia degree [4]. However, it is important to note that due to myopia it is important to note that any intervention may vary from individual to individual due to the diversity of factors affecting myopia. Despite the use of the OK lens, there are still some children with poor control [5].

At present, another method that has been clinically recognized as effective in controlling myopia progression is atropine eye drops. Atropine is a non-selective M-blocker with dose-dependent tolerance, and the higher the concentration, the better the control effect. However, the adverse reactions of high-concentration atropine and the side effects of myopic regression after withdrawal of atropine have limited its wide clinical application to varying degrees [6, 7]. Previous studies by Yam et al. [8] evaluated the efficacy and safety of 0.05%, 0.025%, and 0.01% atropine eye solution and placebo in 1 year. Among the three concentrations used, 0.05% atropine was the most effective in controlling spherical equivalent (SE) and axial length (AL) and the side effects were still acceptable. Therefore, the trend of using 0.05% atropine eye drops to control myopia is becoming more and more obvious. However, many previous studies at domestic and foreign are about the control effect observation of OK lens combined with 0.01% atropine, which leads to a question, that is, the effectiveness and safety analysis of 0.05% combined with OK lens in children with progressive myopia.

2. Atropine eye solution

2.1 Mechanism of atropine eye solution

Atropine is a non-selective muscarinic receptor (M receptor) antagonist. The mechanism of atropine delaying myopia progression has not yet been fully clarified. Currently, the main possible mechanisms are considered as follows: ① Receptor theory: After further destroying the activities of amacrine (M cholinergic receptor) and cholinesterase in the retina, it was found that atropine could still inhibit new sense deprivation myopia. Therefore, atropine may inhibit the deepening of myopia by antagonizing M receptors in choroid or sclera, reducing eye overregulation by relieving smooth muscle spasm, and inhibiting vitreous prolongation. In addition, atropine can directly act on the M receptors of retina and sclera, and inhibit the remodeling of posterior polar sclera mediated by M1 and M4 receptors, delaying the growth of AL [7]. ② Light theory: After the use of atropine, the pupil dilates, which can increase the retina's acceptance of ultraviolet radiation and increase the secretion of dopamine, thus delaying the growth of the AL. ③ Improve choroidal blood supply: Atropine can improve choroidal blood supply and scleral biomechanical characteristics, promote choroidal thickness increase, and improve myopia fundus sclera relative hypoxia situation, thereby inhibiting the rapid growth of AL (**Figure 1**) [9].

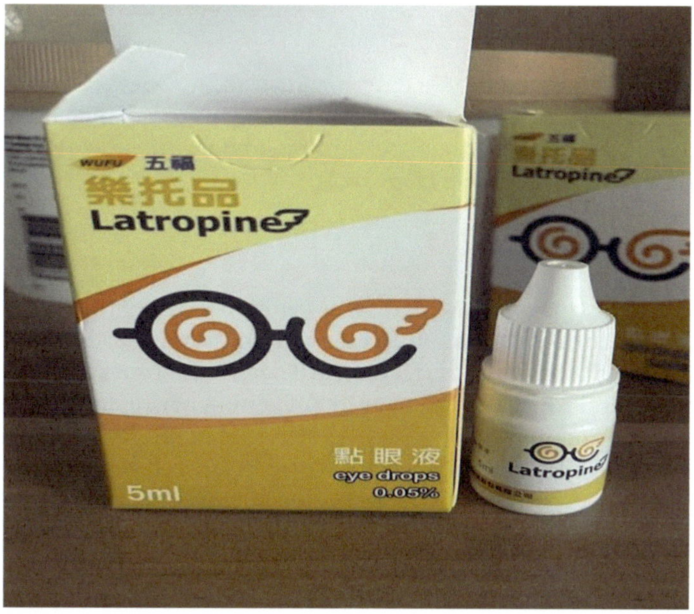

Figure 1.
Atropine eye drops.

2.2 Clinical study of 0.01% and 0.05% atropine for myopia control

Previous studies on atropine in the treatment of myopia (ATOM1) for a period of 2 years have shown that 1% atropine can significantly inhibit myopia progression by about 80% compared with placebo group; however, 1% atropine has significant adverse reactions, such as drug dilation of the pupil, difficulty in seeing near and obvious rebound of myopia after stopping treatment [10]. Therefore, in the ATOM2 study, low concentration of atropine eye solution was studied, and the results showed that 0.5%, 0.1%, and 0.01% atropine eye solution could reduce myopia progression by about 75%, 70%, and 60%, respectively, compared with placebo in the 2-year ATOM1 study. There were almost no significant adverse reactions and rebound effects in the 0.01% atropine group, so the study considered 0.01% atropine to be the most recommended [11]. Since then, clinical reports on atropine have mainly focused on studies of low-concentration atropine. Recently, in the Myopia Progression Control Study (LAMP) conducted by Yam et al. [8], atropine concentrations were 0.05%, 0.025%, and 0.01%. Two-year analysis of SE and AL changes showed that the myopia control effect through low-concentration atropine was significantly better than that of placebo group (0.9% sodium chloride), and the rapid growth of myopia could be effectively controlled by three concentrations of atropine eye drops, and the effect of 0.05% was better. In addition, Moon et al. [12] also found that 0.05%, 0.025%, and 0.01% could effectively inhibit the progression of myopia in Korean children, and the control effect of 0.05% was better than that of the other two. For children whose parents had high myopia and were affected by myopia genetic factors, atropine diluted 0.05% was more suitable. The 1-year SE increase of 0.05%, 0.025%, and 0.01% atropine was −0.27D, −0.46D, and −0.61D, respectively.

3. Orthokeratology (OK)

OK lens is a rigid night-wear high oxygen permeability contact lens, which is currently recognized as one of the effective ways to control myopia, and because of its good myopia-control effect, visual perception, and its safety, reversible advantages have been widely used in the clinic (**Figure 2**).

3.1 Control principle of OK lens

OK lens is a rigid contact lens with reverse geometric design. By wearing it at night, the central corneal curvature is reduced, the cornea is flatted, and the mid-circumference corneal curvature is steepened. The myopia progression is controlled by reducing peripheral retinal hyperfocus or deepening peripheral myopia. A large number of domestic and foreign studies have shown that OK lens can effectively slow down the growth of AL by about 0.15 mm/year, and control the increase of SE by 0.35–0.50D/year [13]. According to the detection of multispectral refraction topography (MRT) in previous studies by Ni et al. [14], the change of retinal hyperfocal amount in children wearing OK lens is significantly smaller than that in the single-vision spectacle lenses group. In addition, in different myopia control treatments, including atropine, defocusing glasses, OK lens, and soft multifocal and bifocal contact lenses, there were significant changes in high-order aberrations, especially the increase of positive spherical aberration and coma, which were significantly negatively correlated with the growth of the AL. The increase of higher-order aberration will significantly inhibit the growth of AL, the development of refractive errors, and the therapeutic effect of myopia control interventions [15–17].

3.2 Factors influencing the control effect of OK lens

Xia et al. [18] found that the width of the outer edge of the defocus ring from the corneal edge produced by wearing OK lenses of different diameters had different effects on controlling and mitigating myopia. The closer the defocus ring was to the corneal edge, the weaker the myopia control effect was. Guo et al. [19] studied and compared the changes of total eye aberrations in children wearing OK lens with a

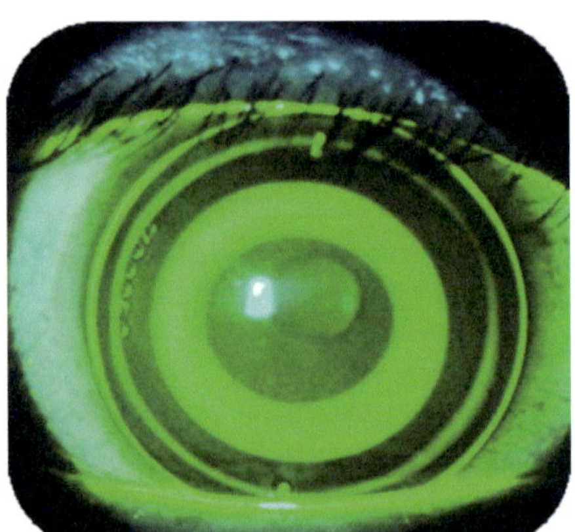

Figure 2.
Orthokeratology.

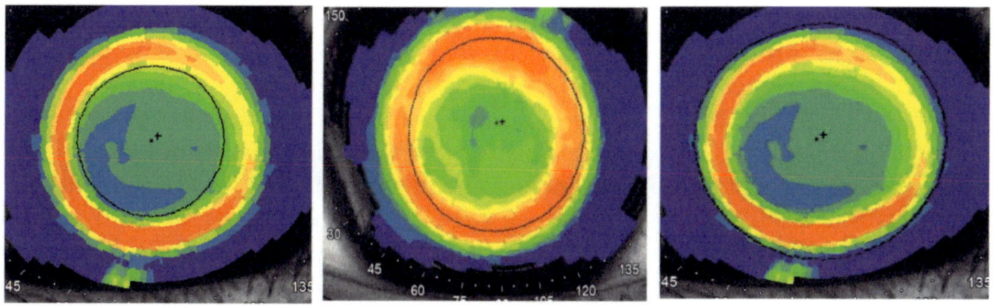

A B C

Figure 3.
A: The defocus ring was outside the pupil. B: The defocus ring matched the pupil. C: The defocus ring was inside the pupil.

back optic zone diameter (BOZD) of 6 mm (6-MM group) and 5 mm (5-MM group) within 2 years and the relationship between them and the elongation of the AL. The results showed that after 2 years, the diameter of the horizontal treatment zone (TZ) in the 5-MM group was less than 1.14 ± 0.11 mm and 6-MM groups, and the axial elongation was less than 0.22 ± 0.07 mm and 6-MM groups. At all follow-up, in total root mean square of higher-order aberrations (HOAs), primary spherical aberration (SA), and coma were also significantly increased in the 5-MM group. However, Paune et al. [20] found that the relative position relationship between the defocus ring and pupil affected the control effect after wearing the OK lens, that is, the control effect was the worst when the defocus ring was outside the pupil and the control effect is medium when the defocus ring was matched the pupil; when the defocus ring was inside the pupil, the control effect is the best, presumably mainly due to enhanced peripheral retinal myopic defocus effect (**Figure 3**).

Previous studies by Chen et al. [21] have shown that larger pupil diameter can help to enhance the control effect of OK lens on delaying axial growth, which is speculated to be mainly due to enhanced defocus effect of peripheral retina myopia. It shows that under different environments, larger pupil can cause more defocus rings to enter the pupil region, thus enhancing the intervention effect of OK lens on peripheral myopic defocus, thus effectively delaying the progression of myopic diopter and AL. In addition, Faria-Ribeiro et al. [22] pointed out that the myopia control effect produced by OK lens may depend on the size of the pupil. Pupil enlargement can increase the illumination of the retina, while more daylight illumination can effectively delay the growth of the AL. In other words, the size of visible pupil and light zone, as well as the relative position relationship between the defocus ring and the pupil zone, are significantly correlated with the myopia control of children wearing the OK lens.

4. Clinical study of low-concentration atropine combined with orthokeratology (OKA) for myopia control

Kinoshita et al. [23] found in a 2-year study in Japan that within 2 years, the AL increased by 0.29 ± 0.20 mm and 0.40 ± 0.23 mm, respectively, in the OK lens combined with 0.01% atropine and in the single OK lens group, where the initial spherical equivalent (SE) of the subject was: −1.00 to −3.00D, the 2-year AL increased by 0.30 ± 0.22 mm and 0.48 ± 0.22 mm, respectively. For subjects with an initial SE of −3.01 to −6.00D, the axial length increased by 0.27 ± 0.15 mm and 0.25 ± 0.17 mm, respectively. Combination therapy was effective in slowing down axial elongation, especially in children with low initial myopia.

Chen et al. [24] conducted a 3-year clinical retrospective study. In the first stage, patients with myopia still increasing rapidly after wearing OK lens and annual axial growth of ≥0.3 mm entered the second stage and were divided into two groups. One group was treated with OK lens combined with 0.01% atropine, and the other group continued to wear OK lens for 2 years. The study results showed that for those with rapid myopia progression and poor control after wearing OK lens, compared with single treatment, 0.01% night atropine combined treatment did not significantly change the 3-year AL elongation results. Wang et al. [25] used a meta-analysis to evaluate the study on the delaying effect of 0.01% atropine combined with OK lens on adolescent myopia. Nine randomized controlled literatures were included after screening, with a total of 858 cases, and the nine literatures were divided into experimental group and control group. The control group was equipped with OK lens alone. The study results showed that compared with OK lens alone, 0.01% atropine combined with OK lens was more effective in controlling the progression of myopia in adolescents.

Wen et al. [26] conducted a 2-year study to explore the control effect of 0.05% atropine combined with OK lens on myopia progression in children. The study subjects were children aged 8–14 with rapid myopia progression. In addition to the use of OK lens, some patients were given 0.05% atropine with low concentration, and the results showed that compared with the OK group, the OKA group showed significantly smaller AL prolongation (0.14 ± 0.13 mm vs. 0.27 ± 0.12 mm). The combination of 0.05% atropine eye drops had a significant effect on 1-year AL prolongation, especially for the control rate of AL in the second half of the year. The results indicated that OK lens combined with 0.05% atropine eye drops could significantly improve the effectiveness of myopia control.

4.1 Factors influencing the control effect of low-concentration atropine combined with orthokeratology (OKA)

Makar et al. [27] found that young age is associated with poor response to treatment with low-concentration atropine. In the concentration studied, young children need the highest concentration of 0.05% to reduce myopia progression, and younger children need a higher concentration of atropine to achieve efficacy similar to that of older children treated with lower concentration. For example, within 2 years, the progress of 10-year-old children in the 0.01% myopia group was similar to that of 8-year-old children in the 0.025% myopia group and similar to that of 6-year-old children in the 0.05% myopia group. This is consistent with the results of Wang et al.'s study [28]. In this study, 90 cases (90 eyes) of progressive myopia patients with 0.34 mm increase in eye axis after 1-year monitoring after wearing OK lenses were selected and randomly divided into two groups; control group 45 eyes were treated with OK lens combined with 0.01% atropine eye solution; 45 eyes in the combination group were treated with OK lens combined with 0.05% atropine eye solution. One year later, the results showed that the AL in the combination group and the control group increased (0.14 ± 0.02 mm vs. 0.25 ± 0.01 mm) compared with before treatment. After treatment, the photopic pupil diameter size increased (2.27 ± 0.10 mm vs. 0.64 ± 0.28 mm) and the mesopic pupil diameter size increased (1.20 ± 0.24 mm vs. 0.38 ± 0.10 mm) in combination group and control group, respectively, compared with that before treatment. After treatment, the relative position relationship between the defocus ring and pupil under photopic pupil in the combination group and the control group changed compared with before treatment. The number of defocus ring smaller than pupil before and after treatment was 18 in the combination group, which was significantly increased compared with 6 before and after treatment, while there was no statistical difference in the control group before and after treatment. These results indicated that OK lens combined with 0.01% and 0.05% atropine could synergically enhance the myopia control effect of adolescents, and especially for young children with rapid myopia degree growth, 0.05% atropine combined with OK lens had a better control effect on progressive myopia.

5. Adverse effects of atropine at low concentration

The main adverse reactions of low-concentration atropine are the inhibition of iris sphincter and ciliary muscle, resulting in decreased eye adjustment, photophobia, and difficulty in vision symptoms.

5.1 Decreased adjustment and pupil reaction

Ha et al. [29] analyzed the effect of 0.01%, 0.02%, 0.025%, 0.05%, 0.1%, 0.25%, 0.5%, and 1% atropine eye drops on myopia control and the performance of adverse reactions, and the results showed that 0.01–1% atropine sulfate eye preparation had control effect on myopia progression. However, the control effect of atropine sulfate is not completely parallel to the concentration, among which 1%, 0.5%, and 0.05% have the same control effect on myopia progression, while the degree of adverse reactions (photophobia and near-vision blur) is related to the concentration, so the low concentration of 0.05% atropine is preferred. In the study by Yam et al. [8], all the low-concentration atropine (0.05%, 0.025%, 0.01%) were well tolerated, and the reduction in the amplitude of adjustment was relatively low in all groups, and only a few subjects required progressive glasses. It is worth noting that the 0.01% atropine group had a similar loss of adaptive ability as the placebo group, and the near vision and optimal correction of hyperopia were not affected in each group. In the study by Fu et al. [30], it was found that 0.02% and 0.01% atropine could reduce the adjustment range by 1.50D and 1.61D, but there was no significant difference between the two concentrations on adjustment and pupil. These studies all showed that low-concentration atropine could lead to decreased adjustment, but most children would not suffer from discomfort. That is to say, the use of atropine at low concentration is relatively safe.

6. Conclusion

The above studies have shown that the effect of low-concentration atropine on myopia control is somewhat concentration-dependent, and it is safe and reliable to use low-concentration atropine in myopia control for young children with rapid myopia progression [31–33]. In addition, the combined use of low concentration atropine and OK lens provides other options to further control the progression of myopia in children, and 0.05% atropine combined with OK lens has a better control effect on progressive myopia [26, 34, 35]. The main mechanism lies in 1. Atropine has concentration-dependent tolerance, and the higher the concentration, the better the control effect [36–39]. 2. About 0.05% atropine has more defocus rings entering the pupil region after pupil enlargement, which enhances the intervention effect of periretinal myopia defocus [40, 41]. 3. Pupil enlargement, higher aberrations of the whole eye, especially positive spherical aberration and coma increase, are significantly negatively correlated with the growth AL, and the increase of higher aberration will significantly inhibit the growth of AL [15–17]. 4. Pupil enlargement can increase retinal illumination, more light enters the fundus, and stimulate the secretion of dopamine [15]. In addition, the adverse reactions after long-term use of low-concentration atropine and whether there is rebound phenomenon after drug withdrawal are still unclear, and these problems need to be supplemented by increasing the sample size in subsequent studies. It is worth noting that for these children who still show progressive myopia after wearing the OK lens in clinic, we choose to provide relevant literature and data support.

Acknowledgements

My sincere thanks to Ling Ai, Benchu Feng, and Zhilong Yang for their great collaborations in the elaboration of this manuscript.

Conflict of interest

I seriously declare that I have no interest whatsoever, only the academic one, in the elaboration of this chapter.

Notes/thanks/other declarations

I express special thanks for the invitation for the collaboration of this chapter and to the authors of the references included in it.

Author details

Duo Xu[1*], Yunyun Wang[1], Ling Ai[2], Benchu Feng[2], Zhilong Yang[3] and Fuliang Li[4]

1 Chongqing Wodi Ophthalmology, Chongqing, China

2 Chongqing Nanping Aier Eye Hospital, Chongqing, China

3 National Open University, Sichuan, China

4 Chongqing He's Eye Hospital, Chongqing, China

*Address all correspondence to: xd15123230263@163.com

References

[1] Holden BA, Fricke TR, Wilson DA, et al. Global prevalence of myopia and high myopia and temporal trends from 2000 through 2050. Ophthalmology. 2016;**123**(5):1036-1042. DOI: 10.1016/j.ophtha.2016.01.006. Epub 2016 Feb 11

[2] Xu X, He XG. Strengthening the understanding of the pathological evolution of myopia. Zhonghua Yan Ke Za Zhi. 2019;**55**(10):721-725. Chinese. DOI: 10.3760/cma.j.issn.0412-4081.2019.10.001

[3] Huang J, Wen D, Wang Q, et al. Efficacy comparison of 16 interventions for myopia control in children: A network meta-analysis. Ophthalmology. 2016;**123**(4):697-708. DOI: 10.1016/j.ophtha.2015.11.010. Epub 2016 Jan 27

[4] Bullimore MA, Johnson LA. Overnight OK lens. Contact Lens & Anterior Eye. 2020;**43**(4):322-332. DOI: 10.1016/j.carolcarrolllae2020.03.018. Epub 2020 Apr 22

[5] Cho P, Cheung SW. Retardation of myopia in OK lens (ROMIO) study: A 2-year randomized clinical trial. Investigative Ophthalmology & Visual Science. 2012;**53**(11):7077-7085. DOI: 10.1167/iovs.12-10565

[6] Chia A, Lu QS, Tan D. Five-year clinical trial on atropine for the treatment of myopia 2: Myopia control with atropine 0.01% eyedrops. Ophthalmology. 2016;**123**(2):391-399. DOI: 10.1016/j.ophtha.2015.07.004. Epub 2015 Aug 11

[7] Upadhyay A, Beuerman RW. Biological mechanisms of atropine control of myopia. Eye & Contact Lens. 2020;**46**(3):129-135. DOI: 10.1097/ICL.0000000000000677

[8] Yam JC, Jiang Y, Tang SM, Law AK, Chan JJ, Wong E, et al. Low-concentration atropine for myopia progression (LAMP) study: A randomized, double-blinded, placebo-controlled trial of 0.05%, 0.025%, and 0.01% atropine eye drops in myopia control. Ophthalmology. 2019;**126**(1):113-124

[9] Zhou X, Zhang S, Zhang G, Chen Y, Lei Y, Xiang J, et al. Increased choroidal blood perfusion can inhibit form deprivation myopia in Guinea pigs. Investigative Ophthalmology & Visual Science. 2020;**61**(13):25. DOI: 10.1167/iovs.61.13.25

[10] Chua WH, Balakrishnan V, Chan YH, et al. Atropine for the treatment of childhood myopia. Ophthalmology. 2006;**113**(12):2285-2291

[11] Chia A, Chua WH, Wen L, et al. Atropine for the treatment of childhood myopia: Changes after stopping atropine 0.01%, 0.1% and 0.5%. American Journal of Ophthalmology. 2014;**157**(2):451-457.e1

[12] Moon JS, Shin SY. The diluted atropine for inhibition of myopia progression in Korean children. International Journal of Ophthalmology. 2018;**11**(10):1657-1662

[13] Li SM, Kang MT, Wu SS, et al. Efficacy, safety and acceptability of OK lens on slowing axial elongation in myopic children by meta-analysis. Current Eye Research. 2016;**41**(5):600-608. DOI: 10.3109/02713683.2015.1050743. Epub 2015 Aug 3

[14] Ni NJ, Ma FY, Wu XM, Liu X, Zhang HY, Yu YF, et al. Novel application of multispectral refraction topography in the observation of myopic control effect

by OK lens in adolescents. World Journal of Clinical Cases. 2021;**9**(30):8985-8998. DOI: 10.12998/WJCCv9.I30.8985

[15] Hughes RP, Vincent SJ, Read SA, Collins MJ. Higher order aberrations, refractive error development and myopia control: A review. Clinical & Experimental Optometry. 2020;**103**(1):68-85. DOI: 10.1111/cxo.12960. Epub 2019 Sep 6

[16] Vincent SJ, Tan Q, Ng ALK, et al. Higher order aberrations and axial elongation in combined 0.01% atropine with OK lens for myopia control. Ophthalmic and Physiological Optics. 2020;**40**(6):728-737

[17] Lau JK, Vincent SJ, Cheung SW, Cho P. The influence of OK lens compression factor on ocular higher-order aberrations. Clinical & Experimental Optometry. 2020;**103**(1):123-128. DOI: 10.1111/cxo.12933. Epub 2019 Jul 1

[18] Guoxuan X, Shaohua W, Lin W, et al. Influence of distance from focal ring to corneal limbal width on myopia control after wearing OK lens. International Journal of Ophthalmology. 2019;**19**(1):3. DOI: 10.3980/j.issn.1672-5123.2019.1.26

[19] Guo B, Cho P, Cheung SW, Kojima R, Vincent S. Optical changes and association with axial elongation in children wearing OK lens lenses of different back optic zone diameter. Eye and Vision. 2023;**10**(1):25. DOI: 10.1186/s40662-023-00344-3

[20] Paune J, Fonts S, Rodriguez L, Queiros A. The role of back optic zone diameter in myopia control with OK lens lenses. Journal of Clinical Medicine. 2021;**10**(2):336

[21] Chen Z, Niu L, Xue F, Qu X, Zhou Z, Zhou X, et al. Impact of pupil diameter on axial growth in OK lens. Optometry and Vision Science. 2012;**89**(11):1636-1640. DOI: 10.1097/OPX.0b013e31826c1831

[22] Faria-Ribeiro M, Navarro R, Gonzalez-Meijome JM. Effect of pupil size on wavefront refraction during OK lens. Optometry and Vision Science. 2016;**93**(11):1399-1408. DOI: 10.1097/OPX.0000000000000989

[23] Kinoshita N, Konno Y, Hamada N, Kanda Y, Shimmura-Tomita M, Kaburaki T, et al. Efficacy of combined OK lens and 0.01% atropine solution for slowing axial elongation in children with myopia: A 2-year randomised trial. Scientific Reports. 2020;**10**(1):12750. DOI: 10.1038/s41598-020-69710-8

[24] Chen Z, Zhou J, Xue F, Qu X, Zhou X. Two-year add-on effect of using low concentration atropine in poor responders of OK lens in myopic children. The British Journal of Ophthalmology. 2022;**106**(8):1069-1072. DOI: 10.1136/bjophthalmol-2020-317980. Epub 2021 Mar 11

[25] Wang JY, Gu Tien F, Li SC, et al. Meta-analysis of 0.01% atropine combined with OK lens in delaying myopia progression in adolescents. The Eye Optometry and Vision Science. 2022;**24**(1):6. DOI: 10.3760/cma.J.c.n115909-20210423-00165

[26] Wen L, Liu H, Xu Q, et al. Add-on effect of using 0.05% atropine in fast progressors of orthokeratology: A preliminary retrospective study[J]. Contact Lens and Anterior Eye. 2025;**48**(1). DOI: 10.1016/j.clae.2024.102282

[27] Makar AB, McMartin KE, Palese M, Tephly TR. Formate assay in body fluids: Application in methanol poisoning. Biochemical Medicine.

1975;**13**(2):117-126. DOI: 10.1016/0006-2944(75)90147-7

[28] Wang YY, Da Z, Ai L, et al. A regulatory synergistic effect of 0.05% atropine combined with OK lens lenses on the defocus ring in progressive myopia. Chinese Journal of Optometry and Vision Science. 2023;**25**(12):913-919. DOI: 10.3760/cma.j.cn115909-20230410-00105

[29] Ha A, Kim SJ, Shim SR, Kim YK, Jung JH. Efficacy and safety of 8 atropine concentrations for myopia control in children: A network meta-analysis. Ophthalmology. 2022;**129**(3):322-333. DOI: 10.1016/j.ophtha.2021.10.016. Epub 2021 Oct 22

[30] Fu A, Stapleton F, Wei L, Wang W, Zhao B, Watt K, et al. Effect of low-dose atropine on myopia progression, pupil diameter and accommodative amplitude: Low-dose atropine and myopia progression. The British Journal of Ophthalmology. 2020;**104**(11):1535-1541. DOI: 10.1136/bjophthalmol-2019-315440. Epub 2020 Feb 21

[31] Yang N, Bai J, Liu L. Low concentration atropine combined with OK lens in the treatment of axial elongation in children with myopia: A meta-analysis. European Journal of Ophthalmology. 2022;**32**(1):221-228. DOI: 10.1177/1120672121998903. Epub 2021 Mar 7

[32] Wang Z, Wang P, Jiang B, Meng Y, Qie S, Yan Z. The efficacy and safety of 0.01% atropine alone or combined with OK lens for children with myopia: A meta-analysis. PLoS ONE. 2023;**18**(7):e0282286. DOI: 10.1371/journalpone.0282286

[33] Tan Q, Ng AL, Cheng GP, Woo VC, Cho P. Combined 0.01% atropine with OK lens in childhood myopia control (AOK) study: A 2-year randomized clinical trial. Contact Lens & Anterior Eye. 2023;**46**(1):101723. DOI: 10.1016/j.carolcarrolllae.2022.101723. Epub May 31 2022

[34] Zambrano Peralta P, Ortiz Quito M, Guerrero Ortiz F, Cervantes AL. OK lens vs. OK lens combined with atropine for the control of myopia in children: Systematic review. Archivos de la Sociedad Española de Oftalmología (English Edition). 2023;**98**(10):568-576. DOI: 10.1016/j.oftale.2023.08.001. Epub 2023 Aug 22

[35] Tsai WS, Wang JH, Chiu CJ. A comparative study of OK lens and low-dose atropine for the treatment of anisomyopia in children. Scientific Reports. 2020;**10**(1):14176. DOI: 10.1038/s41598-020-71142-3

[36] Prousali E, Haidich AB, Fontalis A, Ziakas N, Brazitikos P, Mataftsi A. Efficacy and safety of interventions to control myopia progression in children: An overview of systematic reviews and meta-analyses. BMC Ophthalmology. 2019;**19**(1):106. DOI: 10.1186/s12886-019-1112-3

[37] Wu PC, Chuang MN, Choi J, et al. Update in myopia and treatment strategy of atropine use in myopia control. Eye. 2019;**33**(1):3-13

[38] Chierigo A, Ferro Desideri L, Traverso CE, Vagge A. The role of atropine in preventing myopia progression: An update. Pharmaceutics. 2022;**14**(5):900. DOI: 10.3390/pharmaceutics14050900

[39] Li FF, Yam JC. Low-concentration atropine eye drops for myopia progression. Asia-Pacific Journal of Ophthalmology (Philadelphia, PA.). 2019;**8**(5):360-365. DOI: 10.1097/APO.0000000000000256

[40] Smith EL 3rd. Prentice Award Lecture 2010: A case for peripheral optical treatment strategies for myopia. Optometry and Vision Science. 2011;**88**(9):1029-1044. DOI: 10.1097/OPX.0b013e3182279cfa

[41] Hu HL, Li SZ, Feng AY, Zhong HX, Mu JF, Liu MZ. Relative peripheral refraction in school children with different refractive errors using a novel multispectral refraction topographer. International Journal of Ophthalmology. 2024;**17**(8):1477-1482. DOI: 10.18240/ijo.2024.08.13